SOMATIC EXERCISES FOR BEGINNERS

Release Stress, Find Peace, and Reclaim Your Wellbeing with Gentle Movement

Charles K Benavides

TABLE OF CONTENT

HOW TO SCAN QR CODE

To scan a QR code, take the following general actions:

1. Open the Camera App: The majority of contemporary smartphones come with a built-in QR code scanning feature in their camera apps. Open the camera app on your smartphone.

2. Set the Camera Position: Slightly shake your phone and aim the camera toward the QR code you wish to scan. Verify that the well-lit QR code is inside the frame.

3. Scan the QR Code: The QR code ought to be instantly recognized by your smartphone's camera app. It could provide a link or a notification to access the content linked to the QR code.

4. Follow the Prompt: After the QR code is detected, adhere to any on-screen instructions. This could include clicking on a link to visit a website, downloading an application, or seeing particular content.

5. Access the Content : You ought to be able to view the content linked to the QR code after scanning it and following any instructions. This might be a website, an electronic voucher, contact details, or other kinds of information.

You might need to enable the QR code recognition option in your smartphone's settings or download a QR code scanning app from the app store if the camera app on your phone isn't picking up codes automatically. You should consult your device's user manual for more details since certain devices might have unique motions or instructions for reading QR codes.

INTRODUCTION

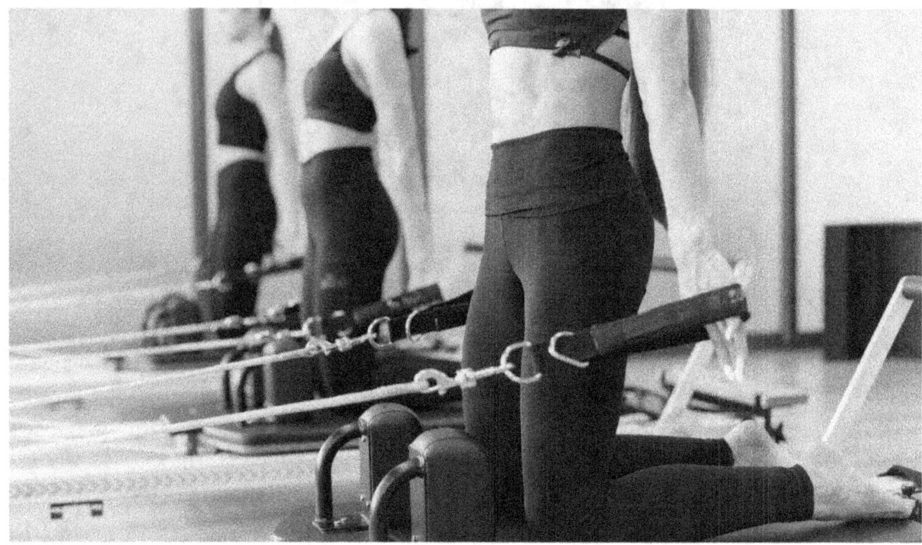

Somatics has become a powerful tool in the quest for holistic well-being, helping to better understand and enhance the mind-body relationship. This book provides a basic overview of the concepts and methods of somatics, acting as a gateway to the field.

Comprehending Somatics

The term "soma" (from the Greek "soma," which means "body") refers to a holistic approach to health that recognizes the interconnectedness of thoughts, feelings, and physical experiences. Fundamentally, somatics acknowledges that our mental and emotional moods can have a significant impact on our physical experiences and motions, and vice versa.

1. The Link Between Mind and Body: We examine the complex interrelationships between the mind and body and how ideas, feelings, and physical experiences interact to influence our general state of well-being. We disentangle the connections between mind and body, ranging from the effects of stress on physical health to the function of movement in emotional regulation.

2. Consciousness in Body: The development of embodied awareness—the capacity to tune into and completely live our bodily sensations and experiences—is essential to somatic

activities. Somatic practices and attentive attention can help people become more aware of their bodies, which can lead to improved self-awareness and self-control.

3. omatic Education Foundations: We examine ideas like pandiculation, sensory-motor learning, and the nervous system's function in somatic processing as we delve into the fundamental ideas of somatic education. Gaining an understanding of these ideas is the first step towards carrying out somatic practices purposefully and successfully.

4. Advantages of Somatic Activities: Somatic activities offer a wide range of advantages for overall well-being, from improving movement efficiency and fostering emotional resilience to relieving chronic pain and lowering stress. We look at the data demonstrating the efficacy of somatic therapies across a range of wellness and health domains.

5. Including Somatics in Everyday Life: We wrap up our investigation of somatics by talking about useful methods for applying somatic concepts to daily life. People can use somatics to build more vitality and presence in their daily experiences, whether through guided moments of embodied awareness, mindful movement activities, or basic mindfulness exercises.

What Are Somatic Exercises?

Somatic exercises are a kind of moderate physical activity that helps people become more aware of their bodies, relax their muscles, and move more efficiently. Somatic exercises emphasize paying careful attention to body sensations and movement patterns, in contrast to standard exercise regimens that only emphasize physical intensity.

Important components of somatic training consist of:

1. Somatic exercises are mindful movements that are done slowly and deliberately while paying close attention to body sensations. People can improve their kinesthetic intelligence (the capacity to perceive and regulate bodily movements) and proprioception (the feeling of body position) by developing a conscious awareness of movement.

2. Increased awareness of the body's sensory feedback, such as tension, relaxation, warmth, and proprioception, is fostered by somatic exercises. Individuals can detect areas of muscular stress or imbalance and undertake corrective motions to restore optimal function by tuning into these sensory cues.

3. A key component of somatic workouts is pandiculation, which is the three-step contraction, release, and relaxation of specific muscle groups. Individuals can facilitate more ease and freedom of movement by resetting typical patterns of muscular contraction through pandiculation.

4. Neuroplasticity: The brain's ability to rearrange neural connections in response to experience is a feature that somatic workouts capitalize on. People can promote brain changes that support better motor control, coordination, and proprioception by practicing conscious, repetitive movement.

Somatic activities provide an embodied and attentive way to improve mental, emotional, and physical health. Somatic exercises help people develop more self-awareness, resilience, and vitality by combining the concepts of mindfulness, sensory awareness, and neuroplasticity.

The Mind-Body Link

The complex interrelationship between mental functions, emotional emotions, and physical sensations is known as the "mind-body connection." This is a succinct examination of the main ideas surrounding the mind-body connection:

1. Psychophysiological Interactions: A complex web of neuronal, hormonal, and metabolic channels facilitates bidirectional communication between the mind and body. Bodily sensations and experiences can shape cognitive processes and emotional states, whereas psychological elements like stress, emotions, and beliefs can affect physiological functions including heart rate, blood pressure, and immunological response.

2. The stress response, also referred to as the "fight-or-flight" response, is a series of physiological reactions that include tense muscles, rapid heartbeat, and shallow respiration. Chronic stress underscores the significant influence of psychological stress on physical health by being linked to a host of health problems such as immunological dysfunction, musculoskeletal discomfort, and hypertension.

3. Emotional Regulation: The body is an important emotional regulator; feelings and motions within the body are potent indicators of emotional states. Through the development of a mindful awareness of one's own body and the encouragement of relaxation responses, mind-body activities like yoga, mindfulness meditation, and somatic exercises provide useful techniques for controlling emotions.

4. Embodied Cognition: According to the embodied cognition theory, interactions with the environment and body sensations serve as the foundation for cognitive processes. Embodied cognition emphasizes the interdependent relationship between body and mind in forming our ideas, perceptions, and behaviors, from the impact of posture on mood and decision-making to the function of gestures in language understanding.

The mind-body link emphasizes how psychological and physiological processes interact profoundly, influencing how we perceive health, sickness, and overall well-being. People can leverage the capacity of embodied cognition and psychophysiological self-regulation to support resilience and holistic health by developing a mindful awareness of the mind-body link.

Benefits of Somatic Practices

Somatic practices are a vital tool for improving overall quality of life since they have so many positive effects on mental, emotional, and physical health. Let's examine the wide range of advantages that somatic practices can offer:

1. Pain Reduction and Injury Recovery: Somatic therapies are well known for their ability to reduce persistent pain and aid in injury recovery. Somatic exercises can help people with back discomfort, neck tightness, and stiff joints by focusing on muscle tension, adjusting posture, and increasing movement efficiency.

2. Relaxation and Stress Reduction: Stress is a common problem that affects both physical and mental health in today's fast-paced society. Through the promotion of relaxation responses, the soothing of the nervous system, and the cultivation of conscious awareness of bodily sensations, somatic activities offer effective methods for stress reduction. People can relax, de-stress, and regain a sense of equilibrium and calm by using methods including deep breathing, gradual relaxation, and gentle movements.

3. Better Movement and Flexibility: Somatic exercises help people move more easily and fluidly by improving their movement efficiency, coordination, and flexibility. Somatic practices can improve physical performance in a variety of activities and sports, assist people overcome restrictions, lower their risk of injury, release muscle tension, and improve joint mobility while also retraining movement patterns.

4. Increased Mindfulness and Body Awareness: Somatic activities develop a more acute awareness of the sensations, motions, and postures of the body, which promotes increased self-control and mindfulness. People can gain a deeper understanding of their bodies, emotions, and inner experiences by tuning into the present moment with curiosity and nonjudgmental awareness. This can increase resilience, emotional intelligence, and self-awareness.

5. Emotional Regulation and Well-Being: Somatic practices place a strong emphasis on the mind-body connection and employ strategies to control emotions and enhance emotional well-being. Somatic techniques generate a stronger sense of peace, clarity, and emotional balance while helping people manage stress, anxiety, and depression by encouraging relaxation responses and conscious awareness of body sensations.

CHAPTER 1

SOMATIC EXERCISES AS A BASIS FOR DEVELOPING BODY AWARENESS

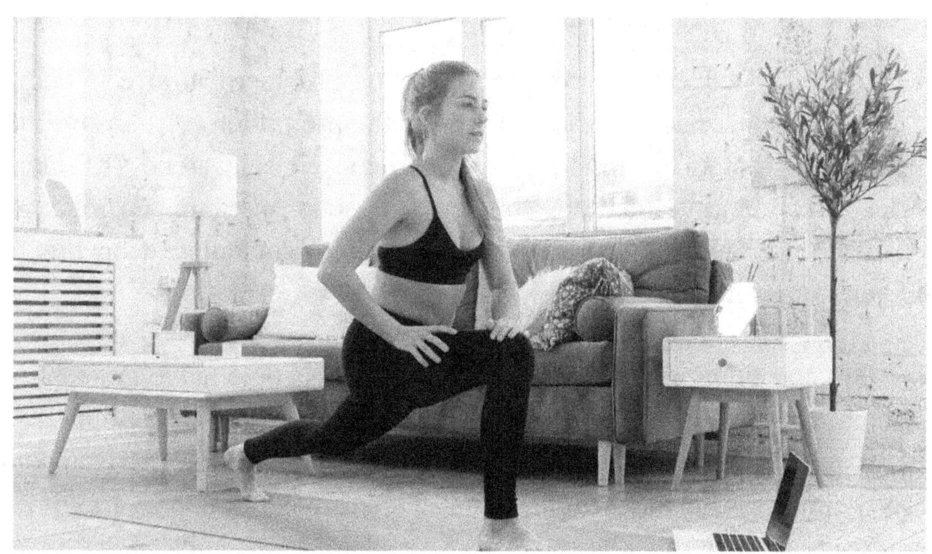

Cultivating bodily awareness is a fundamental component of somatic practices that contribute to the pursuit of holistic wellness. This article examines the importance of growing body awareness and provides helpful advice on how people might pay careful attention to their body sensations to enhance their somatic experience:

1. Comprehending Body Awareness: The capacity to tune into and fully embody the body's sensations, movements, and postural patterns is referred to as body awareness. It entails developing proprioceptive feedback, careful attention to body sensations, and an understanding of how ideas, feelings, and physical experiences interact.

2. The advantages of body awareness Gaining an understanding of one's body has numerous advantages for one's mental, emotional, and physical health. Through the ability to tune into their body's sensations, people can pinpoint areas of tension, imbalance, or discomfort and then start making the necessary corrections to get back to optimal performance. Furthermore, body awareness promotes increased self-control, emotional stability, and mindfulness, enabling people to face obstacles in life more gracefully and fully.

3. Fundamentals of Self-Awareness The concepts of mindfulness, sensory awareness, and embodied cognition serve as the foundation for body awareness. It entails learning to pay attention to physical sensations without passing judgment, investigating movement with curiosity and openness, and seeing how closely the mind and body are intertwined in forming our subjective experiences.

4. Methods for Raising Your Body Awareness: Numerous methods for improving sensory-motor integration and body awareness can be found in somatic exercises. Body scanning exercises, breath awareness exercises, mild movement explorations, and guided relaxation techniques are a few examples of these. Through the purposeful and mindful application of these activities, people can enhance their somatic experience and promote greater embodiment.

5. Embodied Inquiry: People can develop a closer relationship with their bodies and discover new realms of movement, sensation, and self-expression by starting an embodied exploration journey. Somatic techniques, such as the Feldenkrais Method, Alexander Technique, and Body-Mind Centering, help people become more adept at moving with greater ease and flexibility, develop their kinesthetic intelligence, and find renewed ease and liberation in their bodies.

6. Including Body Awareness in Everyday Activities: Developing body awareness goes beyond formal somatic exercises and includes incorporating sensory awareness and mindful movement into daily tasks. People can enhance their somatic experience and promote general well-being by mindfully paying attention to posture, breath, and movement in their everyday routines, whether they are walking, sitting at a computer, or doing home chores.

Cultivating bodily awareness is the cornerstone of somatic practices, providing access to increased vitality, presence, and embodied well-being. People can awaken to the richness of embodied living and enhance their somatic experience by practicing focused attention to their bodies and movement patterns.

Methods of Sensory Awareness

By improving our awareness of our physical experiences, sensory awareness practices aim to help us connect with our bodies on a more profound level. A closer look at how these exercises improve somatic awareness is provided below:

1. Focused Attention: Focused attention approaches in sensory awareness ask us to focus on particular parts of the body, like the breath, bodily touch points, or feelings of warmth, tension, or relaxation. By concentrating our attention in this way, we develop more awareness and become more attuned to the minute details of our physical experience.

2. Mindful Observation: Using sensory awareness practices encourages us to pay attention to our bodies with curiosity and without passing judgment. Instead of categorizing feelings as "good" or "bad," we approach them with curiosity and openness, letting them develop and change moment by moment.

3. Embodied Inquiry: By exploring the nature of our physical experience, embodied inquiry is fostered by sensory awareness approaches. Our understanding of our bodies is enhanced and our kinesthetic intelligence is refined when we ask questions like "Where do I feel tension or discomfort in my body?" "How does my breath move through different regions of my torso?" or "What subtle shifts occur in my posture as I transition from sitting to standing?"

4. Integration with Movement: To improve proprioceptive feedback and movement quality, sensory awareness approaches can be combined with movement practices. For instance, we could synchronize movement with breath cycles, investigate changes in movement speed and intensity while being mindful of body sensations, or integrate mindful breathing into yoga asanas.

Procedures for Body Scanning

Body scanning techniques include progressively moving the focus across various body parts, developing a comprehensive awareness of physical sensations, and encouraging self-control and relaxation. The following are some ways that body scanning techniques support somatic inquiry:

1. Progressive Relaxation: Most body scanning techniques start with a methodical muscle group relaxation that works its way up the body to the head and neck. Through the progressive release of tension from various body areas, people can achieve a deeply relaxed state and enhance their physical and mental health.

2. Increased Sensory Awareness: During a body scanning exercise, people move through various body parts, which helps them develop an increased awareness of their own body's feelings. This

can involve tense or uncomfortable spots as well as feelings of warmth, weight, tingling, or pulsation. People can cultivate greater mindfulness and a deeper physical experience by paying attention to these sensations.

3. Self-Regulation and Stress Reduction: Body scanning techniques are effective methods for promoting self-control and lowering stress. Individuals can counteract the physiological impacts of stress, such as higher heart rate, shallow breathing, and muscular tension, by methodically releasing muscle tension and encouraging relaxation responses. In addition, the practice of body scanning activates the parasympathetic nervous system, which helps one achieve a sense of peace.

4. Integration with Mindfulness Meditation: Mindfulness meditation techniques, including loving-kindness meditation or breath awareness, are frequently combined with body scanning procedures. People can develop their somatic awareness, present-moment awareness, acceptance, compassion, and composure by integrating body scanning with mindfulness meditation.

Body scanning exercises and sensory awareness approaches are effective ways to improve somatic awareness and cultivate mindfulness. Through inquiry, openness, and receptivity in these practices, people can develop a deep connection to their bodies, encourage self-regulation and relaxation, and become aware of the richness of embodied living.

Awareness and Control of Breath

1. Breath's Function in Somatic Practices: In somatic exercises, the breath acts as a focus point, opening a portal into the present and promoting the unification of the mind and body. Not only does conscious breathing control physiological processes like blood pressure and heart rate, but it also affects cerebral clarity, emotional states, and general vitality.

2. Consciously Observing Breath: Observing the breath's natural rhythm with conscious attention and impartial awareness is the practice of breath awareness. People can strengthen their bodily experience, ground themselves in the here and now, and develop inner stability and serenity by paying attention to the sensations of inhaling and expiration.

3. Investigating the Soma Using Breath: People can examine the intricate interactions between movement, breath, and body feelings through the medium of somatic exploration. By engaging in techniques like breath-centric movement, diaphragmatic breathing, and mindful breathing, people can improve their proprioceptive feedback, relax, and self-regulate. They can also improve their kinesthetic intelligence.

4. Methods for Controlling Breath: By deliberately adjusting the breath's depth, rhythm, and quality, breath control techniques can affect both psychological and physiological states.

Breathing exercises, rhythmic breathing, deep belly breathing, and alternative nostril breathing are a few examples of these strategies. People can modulate emotional reactivity, regulate the autonomic nervous system, and foster a condition of balance and equilibrium by practicing breath control techniques.

5. Combining Movement Practices with Integration: Movement practices like yoga, tai chi, and somatic movement therapy fluidly incorporate awareness and control of one's breath. These exercises focus on breathing and movement in unison, teaching participants to move when they inhale, relax when they exhale, and develop a smooth and balanced connection between the two. People can improve their somatic awareness, encourage relaxation, and improve proprioception by breathing in time with their movements.

Breath awareness and control are essential components of somatic exercises that provide a means of self-regulation, relaxation, and embodiment. Through the use of breath, people can develop a more profound somatic experience, increase their mindfulness, and set out on a path toward holistic well-being and self-discovery.

FUNDAMENTALS OF MINDFUL MOVEMENT

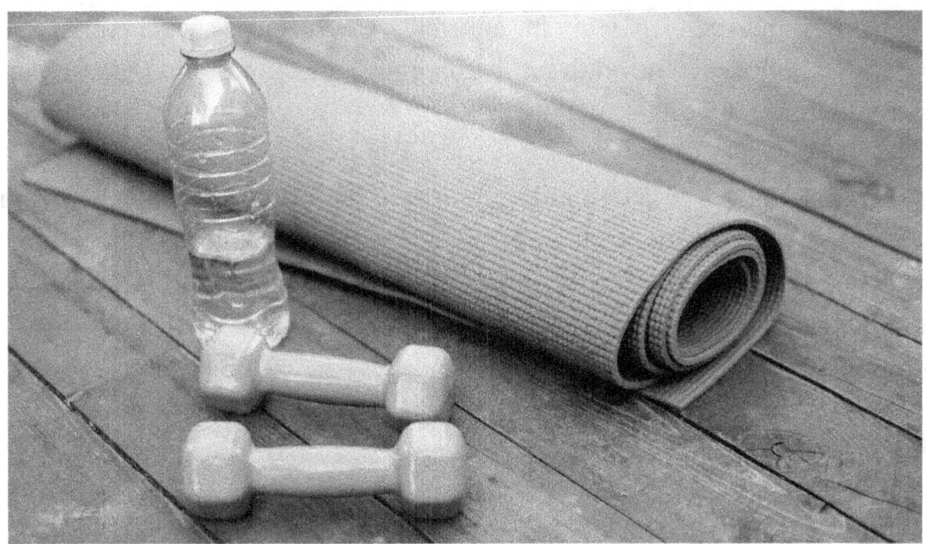

The practice of mindful movement provides a haven of presence and awareness amidst the tumult of modern life. Practicing mindful movement cultivates a strong bond between the mind and body by combining intentionality, mindful attention, and nonjudgmental awareness with physical activity.

Examining Calm Motions

In somatic exercises, gentle movements are a basic technique that encourages people to move with grace, ease, and awareness. Here is a closer examination of the tenets and advantages of investigating soft movements:

1. The Fundamentals of Calm Motions: Instead of using force or rigidity, gentle movements stress attributes of softness, fluidity, and ease. By doing these movements slowly and deliberately, people can learn to pay attention to the finer points of movement and subtle feelings. Gentle movements encourage confidence in the body's inherent wisdom and a sense of safety by emphasizing comfort and relaxation.

2. Paying Close Attention to Feelings: By focusing attention on physical sensations, such as the feeling of joints articulating, the sensation of muscles lengthening and contracting, and the rhythm of breath synchronizing with movement, one can explore mild motions. People can

improve their kinesthetic intelligence and their somatic experience by paying attention to these feelings with inquiry and openness.

3. Inhalation-Based Movement: Soft motions are frequently performed in time with the breath, starting on the inhale and ending on the exhale. This breath-centric method encourages a harmonic connection between movement and breath, as well as relaxation and improved proprioceptive input. People can develop more coherence and fluidity in their somatic experience by synchronizing their breath with movement.

4. Examining Motion Range: In a supportive and safe environment, gentle movements provide an opportunity to explore the entire range of motion of joints and muscles. People are urged to move within their range of comfort to honor their bodies' limitations and prevent strain or discomfort. People can increase their range of motion and enhance their flexibility, mobility, and coordination by progressively doing so.

5. Cautious Stops and Transitions: When you move mindfully, you pay attention to the movements themselves as well as the pauses and transitions between them. These times of change and stillness present important chances for introspection, assimilation, and expanding consciousness. People develop a sense of presence and spaciousness in their dance practice by practicing awareness during transitions and pauses.

6. Advantages of Mild Motions: There are numerous advantages to exploring gentle motions for your emotional, mental, and physical health. Enhanced bodily awareness and proprioception, decreased muscular tension and stiffness, greater joint mobility and flexibility, and elevated relaxation and stress reduction are a few possible advantages. Additionally, gentle motions support a holistic feeling of well-being by encouraging a sense of embodied presence, energy, and inner serenity.

Exploring soft motions is a basic somatic activity that provides an entry point to embodiment, awareness, and overall health. People can develop more somatic awareness, a deeper somatic experience, and a path toward embodied living and self-discovery by doing gentle movements with intentionality and conscious attention.

Fostering Mindfulness While Moving

By encouraging people to move with intentionality and conscious awareness, mindfulness in motion promotes a strong bond between the environment, the body, and the mind. Here is a look at the guidelines and advantages of practicing mindfulness while moving:

1. Awareness of the Present: Anchoring our attention to the present now while maintaining an open-minded curiosity and a non-judgmental awareness of our physical sensations, emotions, and environment is a key component of practicing mindfulness in motion. We can develop a sense of presence and aliveness in our lived experience and enhance our bodily experience by practicing mindfulness in the present moment.

2. Realized Presence: Practicing mindfulness while moving invites us to fully inhabit our bodies and to pay careful attention to and be receptive to the feelings, textures, and rhythms of movement. We can develop a sense of stability, vigor, and groundedness in our movement practice by establishing an embodied presence.

3. With Intention: When we walk with intention and purpose, our movements become more in line with our deepest beliefs and aspirations. This is the invitation to mindfulness in motion. As we investigate the subtleties of feeling, expression, and meaning infused within our movements, each movement becomes a vehicle for self-expression, creativity, and self-discovery.

4. Somatic Investigation: Through the practice of mindfulness in motion, we can go further into our understanding of our bodies, movement patterns, and habitual posture and gesture. This opens the door to somatic investigation. We discover new facets of movement, feeling, and self-expression via attentive observation and investigation, which promotes greater embodiment and kinesthetic intelligence.

5. Combining with Everyday Life: Beyond structured movement exercises, mindfulness in motion encompasses our daily interactions and activities. We can bring mindfulness and presence into our everyday routines, whether we are walking, standing, or doing housework. This will turn normal tasks into chances for bodily inquiry and self-awareness.

Linking Breath and Movement

Breath and movement combined are a potent stimulant for somatic inquiry that enhances our movement practice's flow, coherence, and relaxation. Here are some more details on the benefits and guiding principles of integrating breath and movement:

1. Breath as a Link: Breath connects the rhythm of our internal world with the external world of movement and action, acting as a bridge between the mind and body. We may develop a harmonic relationship between our body and mind and enhance integration, coherence, and flow in our somatic experience by coordinating movement with breath.

2. The ability to coordinate rhythmically: Linking movement and breath entails synchronizing our movement timing and rhythm with our breathing's inherent rhythm. Breath and movement

flow together seamlessly as each movement is started on the inhale and finished on the exhale, improving proprioceptive feedback, encouraging relaxation, and developing a sense of embodied presence.

3. Enhanced Sensitivity: We become more conscious of the complex interactions that exist between breath, movement, and physical feelings when we link movement and breath. In our movement practice, each breath becomes a compass that helps us stay in the present and develops our awareness of the subtleties of movement and sensation.

4. Control of Energy: Breath and movement work together to control the flow of energy in our bodies, fostering harmony, vitality, and balance. Our physiological and psychological moods can be altered by conscious breathing patterns, which can help to promote self-control and relaxation by controlling arousal levels.

5. Development of Presence: In our movement practice, connecting movement with breath fosters a sense of presence and mindfulness, as each breath becomes a doorway to embodied awareness and self-discovery. We can enhance our somatic experience and become more aware of the fullness of embodied existence by focusing on the pattern and quality of our breathing.

Embodied awareness, presence, and integration can be attained through transformative pathways such as practicing mindfulness in motion and integrating movement with breath. By consciously and openly participating in these practices, we develop a deeper somatic experience, increase our self-awareness, and set out on a path toward holistic well-being and self-discovery.

CHAPTER THREE

METHODS OF RELAXATION

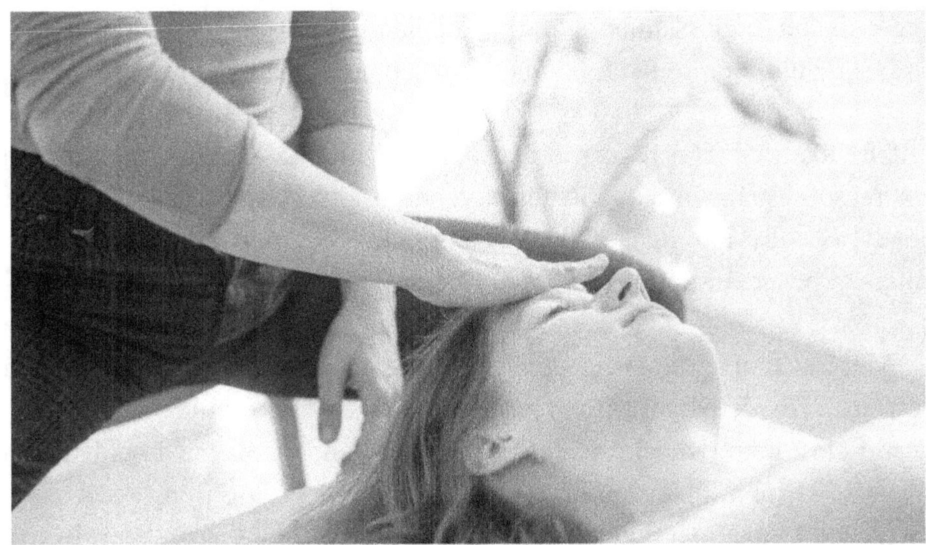

In somatic practices, relaxation techniques are essential because they provide a means of releasing tension, encouraging relaxation, and reestablishing mental and physical balance. Here, we explore the tenets and advantages of Progressive Muscle Relaxation (PMR), a potent technique for stress relief and relaxation:

Gradual Release of Muscle Tension

A methodical relaxation technique called Progressive Muscle Relaxation (PMR) includes tensing and relaxing particular muscle groups to create a deeply relaxed state. Here's a closer look at PMR's guiding ideas and advantages:

1. Theoretical Framework of Progressive Muscle Relaxation The foundation of PMR is the idea that muscle groups should be gradually tense and released, with intervals of relaxation and tension. The method is tensing each muscle group separately for a short while, then letting go of the tension and letting the muscles relax fully. People can encourage relaxation and remove accumulated muscle tension from physical exertion or stress by methodically activating and releasing their tense muscles.

2. Methodical Approach: PMR uses a methodical approach, usually beginning with the feet and working its way up the body to the head and neck muscles. People can methodically release

tension from various muscle groups according to this step-by-step procedure, which encourages a feeling of comfort and relaxation throughout the body.

3. Conscious Awareness: PMR entails developing an attentive awareness of one's body sensations and the dynamic between tension and relaxation. People can develop a deeper somatic experience and a better understanding of the regular patterns of tension and stress contained inside their bodies by tuning into the feelings of muscular tension and release.

4. Response of Relaxation: The relaxation response, which is characterized by a drop in blood pressure, an increase in parasympathetic activity, and a lowered heart rate, is triggered by PMR. PMR counteracts the physiological effects of stress by eliciting a relaxation response, which enhances feelings of peace, tranquility, and well-being.

5. Progressive Muscle Relaxation Advantages: Numerous advantages for mental, emotional, and physical health are provided by PMR. These advantages can include decreased stiffness and tension in the muscles, better sleep, increased resilience and stress management, and a reduction in the symptoms of chronic pain, anxiety, and depression. In addition, PMR encourages inner serenity, renewal, and relaxation, which supports a comprehensive sense of well-being.

6. Real-World Application: People can locate a peaceful, comfortable area to sit or lie down in a relaxed position to practice PMR. People methodically tighten each muscle group for 5–10 seconds, starting with their feet, and then release the tension and let the muscles relax fully for 20–30 seconds. Each muscle group goes through the procedure once more, gradually progressing up the body.

Progressive Muscle Relaxation (PMR) is a powerful relaxation method that provides a straightforward yet efficient means of encouraging calmness, alleviating stress, and enhancing overall well-being. People can develop more inner peace and energy as well as increased relaxation and tension release by including PMR in their everyday practice.

Directed Visualization and Imagery

Using mental images to elicit sensory sensations and encourage healing, relaxation, and stress reduction is known as guided imagery and visualization. A closer examination of the tenets and advantages of guided imagery and visualization is provided below:

1. The fundamentals of guided imagery Through guided visualization, one can conjure up vivid mental images and rich sensory experiences. It consists of audio recordings or guided storytelling that takes users through a sequence of pictures, settings, or situations meant to promote

well-being, relaxation, and tranquility. Guided imagery stimulates the mind-body connection by appealing to the sensations and emotions, which leads to relaxation reactions and promotes healing and self-discovery.

2. Building Cognitive Environments: Through guided imagery, people can construct "mindscapes," or mental landscapes, that provide a peaceful haven for relaxation. These mental landscapes could be imagined places that inspire sentiments of security, coziness, and inner serenity, or peaceful natural locations like beaches, forests, or mountains. People might get a deep sensation of renewal and relaxation by losing themselves in these mental worlds.

3. Improving Perceptual Awareness All of the senses are stimulated by guided imagery, allowing people to see, hear, feel, smell, and even taste the imagined settings or situations. Guided imagery enhances the immersive nature of the experience by stimulating several sense modalities, leading to a profound feeling of awareness and involvement in the present.

4. Reduction of Stress and Healing: It has been demonstrated that guided imagery helps people relax, cope with stress, and lessen the symptoms of anxiety, depression, chronic pain, and other stress-related illnesses. Guided imagery stimulates feelings of well-being and relaxation responses, which in turn trigger the body's healing processes and enhance mental, emotional, and physical health.

5. Goal-Achieving Visualization: By using visualization techniques, one can use their imagination to bring about desired results and accomplish personal objectives. Visualizing oneself accomplishing a certain objective or desired result can help people become more motivated, and confident, and develop a success-oriented attitude.

Restorative Somatic Poses

A simple yet effective technique to reduce tension, encourage relaxation, and bring the body-mind system back into balance is through restorative somatic poses. The concepts and advantages of restorative somatic poses are examined in more detail below:

1. The fundamentals of somatic rehabilitative poses: Assuming cozy, supportive positions that promote deep relaxation and the release of tension in the muscles is the foundation of restorative somatic poses. Usually held for several minutes, these poses enable practitioners to surrender into a deeply restful and rejuvenating condition.

2. Encouraged Calm: Props like blocks, blankets, and bolsters are used in restorative somatic poses to offer comfort and support to the practitioner. People can release muscular strain and

stress by establishing a sense of physical support and containment, which enables the body to fully relax into the pose.

3. Relaxation of Tensed Muscles: Somatic poses that promote restorative alignment help remove built-up muscle tension from physical activity, stress, and extended periods of sitting or standing. Individuals can facilitate a sense of comfort and spaciousness in their bodies by releasing tension from their muscles and connective tissues embracing passive positions and relying on props for support.

4. Relaxation and Stress Reduction: To counteract the physiological consequences of stress and to produce a feeling of calm and tranquility, restorative somatic poses encourage relaxation responses. Restorative poses cause a relaxation response that lowers blood pressure, and heart rate, and improves both physical and mental well-being by stimulating the parasympathetic nerve system.

5. Conscious Awareness: Somatic positions that promote restorative awareness of the body, breath, and mental states. People can develop a sense of inner peace and tranquility as well as a deeper bodily experience by practicing present-moment awareness and nonjudgmental observation.

Restorative somatic poses offer a mild yet effective technique to release tension, promote relaxation, and restore balance to the body-mind system, while guided imagery and visualization offer potent tools for healing, relaxation, and stress reduction. Through the integration of these practices into their everyday regimen, individuals can foster increased resilience, energy, and well-being in their lives.

CHAPTER FOUR

RELEASING TENSION AND STRESS

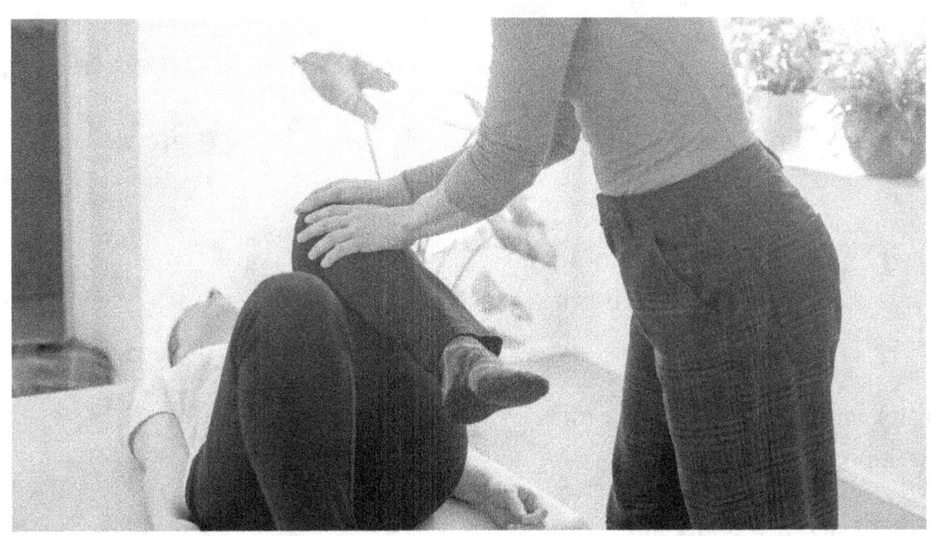

Neck and Shoulder Release

Persistent stress and tension can take many different forms in our bodies, with the neck and shoulders being common places for them to appear. Retaining stress interferes with our ability to move and feel comfortable physically in addition to having an impact on our mental health. To improve general wellness, this article explores somatic exercises that are specifically meant to relieve tension and encourage relaxation in the shoulders and neck.

Somatic Neck and Shoulder Release Benefits

Regular somatic shoulder and neck workouts have the following advantages:

1. Decreased muscle tension: These exercises help ease pain and discomfort by slowly stretching and releasing tight muscles.
2. Enhanced mobility: You can have a greater range of motion and find it simpler to carry out daily tasks if your neck and shoulders are more flexible.
3. Reducing stress: By connecting with your body's reaction to stress, somatic awareness enables you to let go of tension and encourage relaxation.

Somatic Activities for Shoulder and Neck Release

1. Soft Rolls of the Shoulders

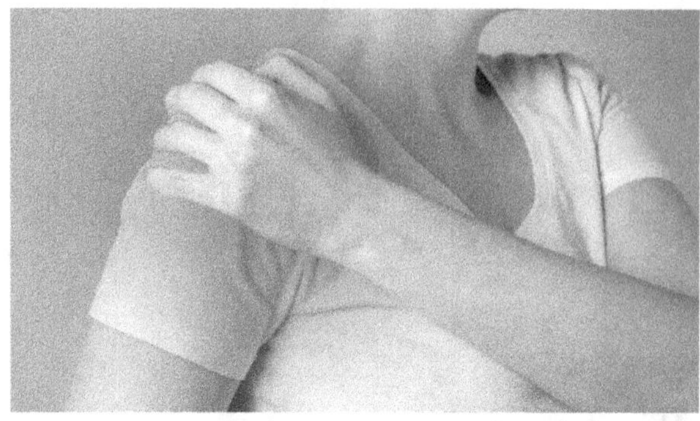

With a lofty stance and relaxed shoulders, sit or stand.

Start by gently moving your shoulders forward in tiny circles while observing how your muscles feel.

Make numerous circles with your shoulders rolled back in the other direction.

Keep an eye out for tense spots and modify your form accordingly.

Five to ten times over, repeat this forward and backward motion.

2. Circles around the neck:

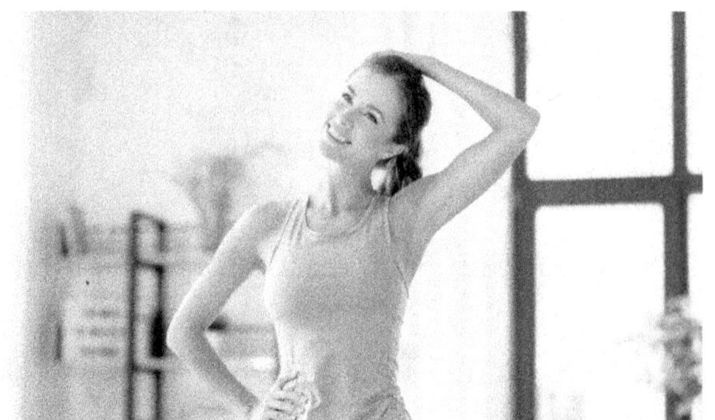

Keep your head up and tuck your chin in when you sit or stand.

Start slowly rotating your head in a clockwise and counterclockwise direction.

Feel the stretch in your neck muscles as you make little, deliberate motions.

Steer clear of any abrupt or violent movements.

Do each direction five to ten times.

3. Bends in the Lateral Neck:

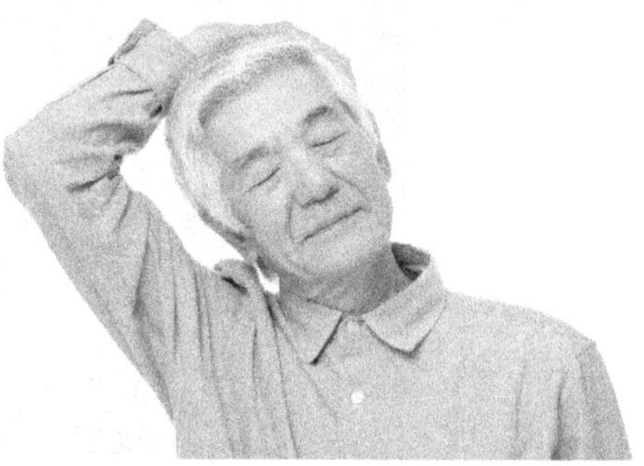

Start with a tall stance while standing or sitting.

Feel the strain down the side of your neck as you slowly incline your ear down towards your shoulder.

Hold for a short while, focusing on any sore spots or regions of tension.

Repeat on the other side after gently bringing your head back to the center.

Make five to ten bends on each side.

4. Head Drop Supported

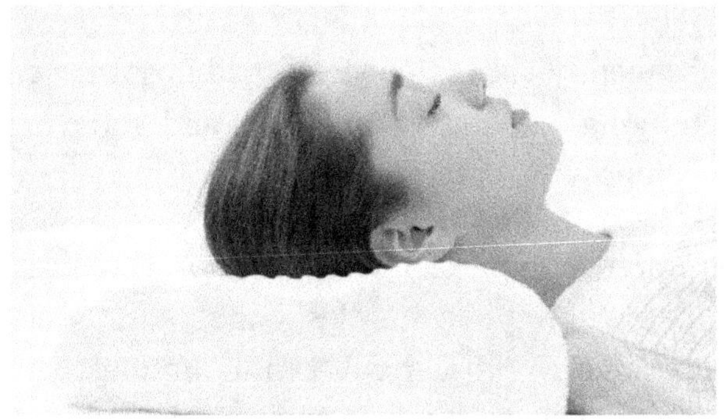

With your knees bent and your feet flat on the ground, take a comfortable position on your back.

Support your head slightly below the base of your skull by placing a bolster or rolled cloth behind your neck.

Release your head and neck weight by allowing it to gently drop back onto the support.

For a few minutes, take deep, slow breaths while paying attention to any feelings in your shoulders and neck.

To exit, softly raise your head back up while slowly contracting your core muscles.

5. Jaw Discharge:

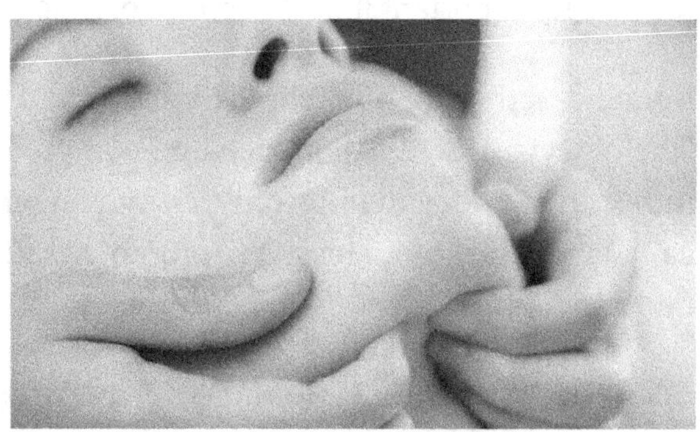

With your shoulders relaxed, take a comfortable seat or stand.

Gently close your mouth and move your lower jaw forward a little, as though you were making a tiny overbite.

For a few seconds, hold, paying attention to any tightness in your jaw muscles.

Bring your jaw back to its neutral position by relaxing it.

Do this five to ten times over.

Bonus Tip: Try combining these somatic exercises with meditation or guided visualization to further improve your relaxation. Visualize your shoulders and neck relaxing and releasing, or see your breath washing away tension with each exhale.

Lower Back Tension and Stress Relief

A common complaint is lower back pain, which is frequently caused by stress, bad posture, and extended periods of sitting. Fortunately, by encouraging attentive movement and relieving tension in important muscle areas, somatic exercises can provide natural relief.

Somatic activities, as previously indicated, focus on interoception, or interior bodily awareness. The objective is to experience and comprehend feelings within your muscles, bones, and tissues rather than concentrating only on movement on the outside. With careful, gentle motions, you can target tense places to promote release and avoid more discomfort thanks to this understanding.

Somatic Lower Back Release's Advantages

Regular lower back somatic exercise practice has the following advantages:

1. Decreased stiffness and pain: Mild stretches and releases help improve lower back muscular flexibility and reduce soreness.
2. Better alignment and general posture can result from releasing tension, which can lessen the load on the lower back.
3. Reducing stress: By connecting with your body's reaction to stress, somatic awareness enables you to let go of tension and encourage relaxation.
4. Enhanced mobility: Your lower back's range of motion can be improved with improved flexibility and release, which will facilitate daily tasks.

Somatic Activities to Relieve Lower Back Pain

Here are three quick and easy somatic exercises that you may perform anywhere:

1. Tilts of the Pelvis:

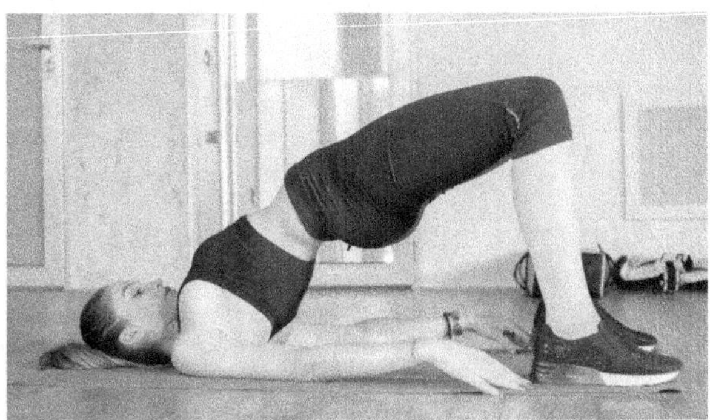

Start by lying on your back with your feet flat on the ground and your knees bent.

Using your core muscles, gently press your lower back into the floor.

Feel for a tiny arch in your lower back as you tilt your pelvis upward.

After a brief period of holding, gradually lower your lower back to the floor.

Do this five to ten times over.

2. Cow-Cat:

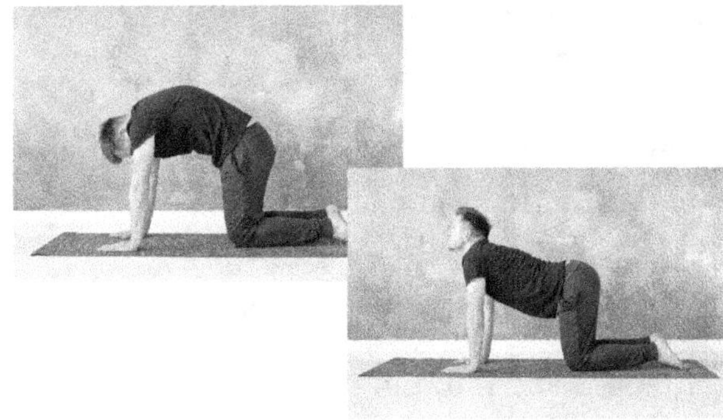

Maintain a neutral spine as you begin on your hands and knees.

Take a deep breath, arch your back like a cat, lower your belly to the floor, and gaze upward.

Breathe out, lowering your chin into your chest, pulling your belly button against your spine, and rounding your back like a cow.

Breathe in sync with your movements, alternating between the cat and cow poses with ease.

Do this five to ten times over.

3. Kneeling and twisting:

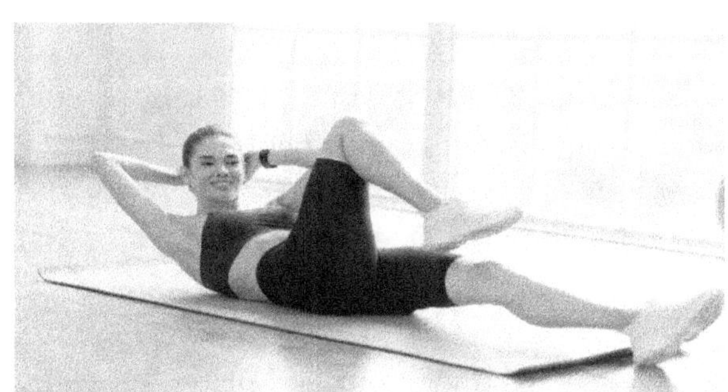

With your feet flat on the ground and your knees bent, lie on your back.

Hugging it with your arms, bring one knee to your chest.

Feel your lower back start to release any tension as you slowly rock from side to side.

Continue on the opposite side.

After you've finished with both knees, bring them both up to your chest and turn them carefully to one side while maintaining your chin tucked in.

After a few breaths of holding, switch to the opposite side.

4. Assisted Child's Position:

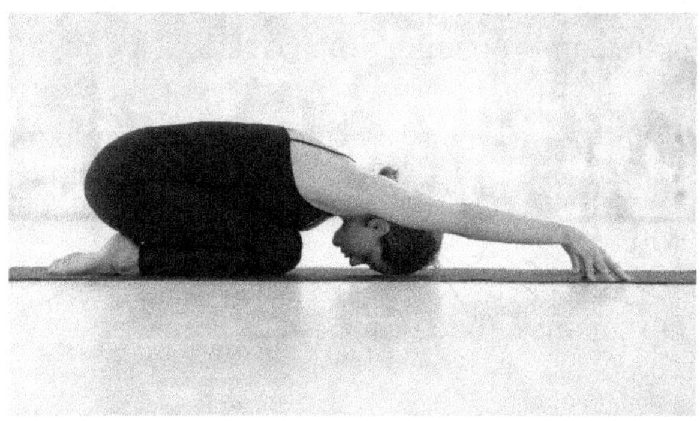

Step onto the floor and start kneeling with your knees hip-width apart and your toes together.

Place your torso between your thighs while you recline back on your heels.

With your palms facing each other or flat, extend your arms forward on the floor.

For extra support, put a bolster or rolled cloth under your forehead.

Lean your shoulders and hips toward the floor and let your body melt into the supported position.

For several minutes, take slow, deep breaths while paying attention to any lower back pain you may feel.

Press your hands into the ground and slowly raise your torso back to a kneeling position to exit.

5. Adapted Figure-Four Extension:

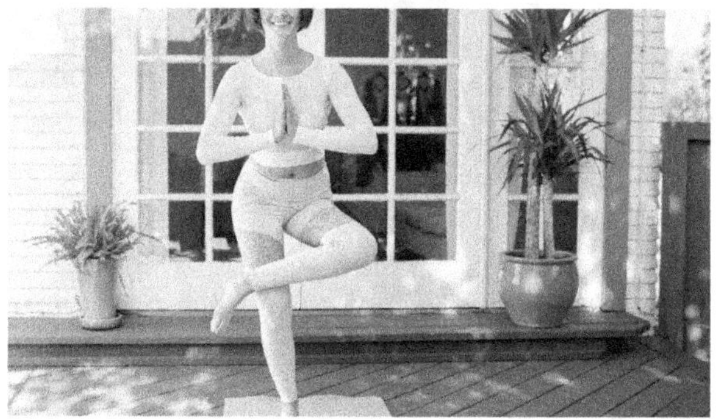

With your feet flat on the floor and both knees bent, take a comfortable position on your back.

Immediately above the knee, cross one ankle across the other thigh.

Wrap your hands gently around the thigh of your elevated leg.

Feel the little stretch in your lower back and glutes as you slowly bring your thigh closer to your chest.

Concentrating on the release in your tense areas, hold for a few breaths.

Continue on the opposite side.

As with all these exercises, keep in mind that gentle stretches and mindful movement should take precedence over any forced motions that result in discomfort. Adjust them to suit your needs, and pay attention to your body's cues.

Hips and Pelvic Floor Relaxation

Although the hips and pelvic floor are frequently disregarded, they are essential for stress management, total body alignment, and stability. Tension stored in these places can cause pain and discomfort, as well as worsen existing conditions like erectile dysfunction or urine incontinence. In these important areas, somatic exercises provide a gentle and efficient means of reducing tension, enhancing mobility, and developing increased awareness and relaxation.

Somatic Hip and Pelvic Floor Relaxation Benefits

Frequent pelvic floor and hip somatic exercises have several advantages:

1. Decreased stiffness and pain: Mild stretches and releases may improve hip and pelvic floor muscle flexibility and reduce soreness.
2. Better pelvic floor function: Relaxing and building these muscles can help with urination as well as infertility.
3. Reducing stress: By connecting with your body's reaction to stress, somatic awareness enables you to let go of tension and encourage relaxation.
4. Improved core stability: Correct posture and core stability are influenced by activating and relaxing the pelvic floor muscles.

Somatic Activities to Promote Pelvic Floor and Hip Relaxation

Here are three quick and easy somatic exercises that you may perform anywhere:

1. Gently rotate your hips:

Place your feet hip-width apart and bend your knees just a little bit.

Start with your hips, carefully tracing little circles in one way at first, then the other.

Instead of putting any tension or force on your movements, concentrate on how your hip joints move.

Do each direction five to ten times.

2. Encouraged Butterfly Stretch:

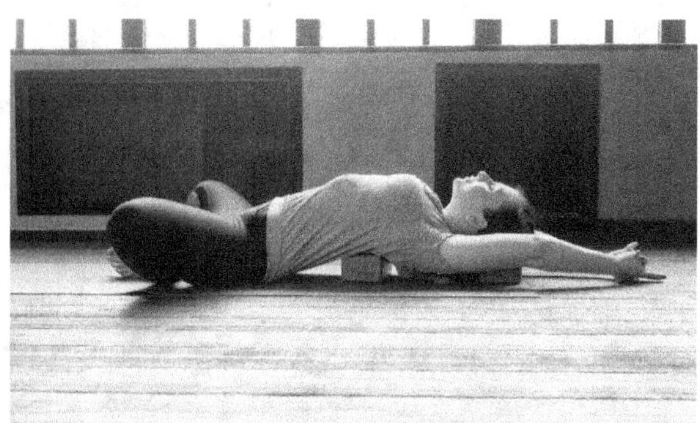

With your feet flat on the ground and your knees bent, lie on your back.

Allowing your knees to naturally fall open, gently bring the soles of your feet together.

For extra support, put a bolster or rolled cloth under your knees.

For a few minutes, take slow, deep breaths while paying attention to any feelings in your pelvic floor and hips.

Press your feet apart slowly and bring your knees back to hip-width apart to exit.

3. Breath on Pelvic Floor:

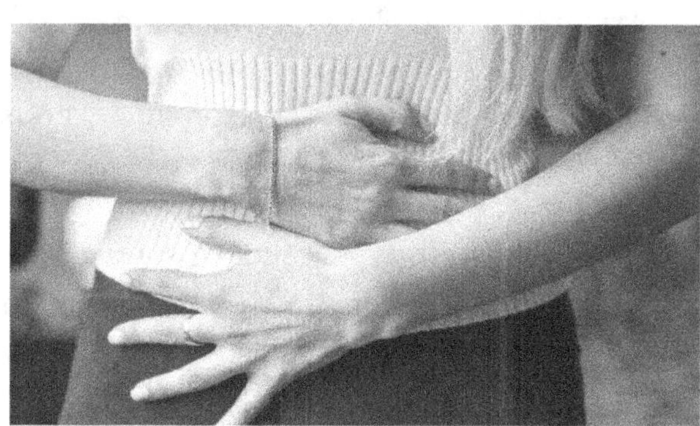

With your feet flat on the ground and your knees bent, lie comfortably on your back.

Put one hand on your stomach and the other, a little above your pubic bone, on your lower abdomen.

Feel your belly gently expand as you take a breath.

Imagine elevating the base of your pelvis as you exhale by pulling your pelvic floor muscles inward and upward.

Pay attention to timing the light pelvic floor contraction with your breath.

Breathe in again and squeeze five to ten times.

4. Stretching in Figure Four while inhaling:

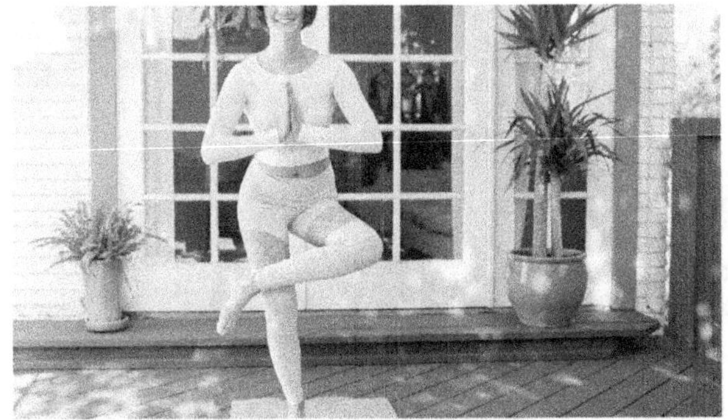

With your feet flat on the floor and both knees bent, take a comfortable position on your back.

Immediately above the knee, cross one ankle across the other thigh.

Wrap your hands gently around the thigh of your elevated leg.

Breathe in, letting go of any tension in your lower back and relaxing your hips.

Imagine elevating the base of your pelvis as you exhale by pulling your pelvic floor muscles inward and upward.

For a few breaths, hold the pose while paying attention to the gradual stretch and synchronized breathing.

Continue on the opposite side.

5. Supported Bridge with Activation of the Pelvic Floor:

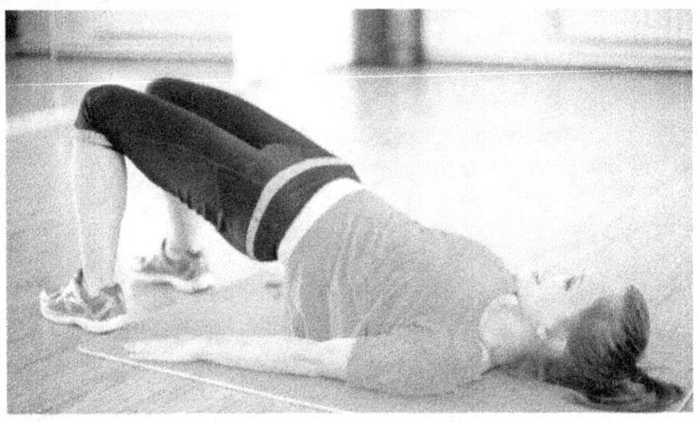

Lay flat on your back with your feet hip-width apart and your knees bent.

For support, place a bolster or rolled towel just above your hips beneath your lower back.

Forming a bridge, slowly raise your hips off the ground while firmly pressing your feet into the floor.

Lift and hold your pelvic floor muscles gently as you approach the top of the bridge.

For a few breaths, breathe slowly and deeply while keeping your pelvic floor activated.

With a slow and deliberate movement, return your hips to the floor while relaxing your pelvic floor muscles.

Five to ten times over

Bonus Tip: Try combining these exercises with guided visualizations that emphasize releasing tension and fostering peace in your pelvic floor and hips to further enhance your relaxation experience. Visualize a warm light stream covering these regions, easing and dissipating any tension.

CHAPTER FIVE

POSTURE AND ALIGNMENT IMPROVEMENT

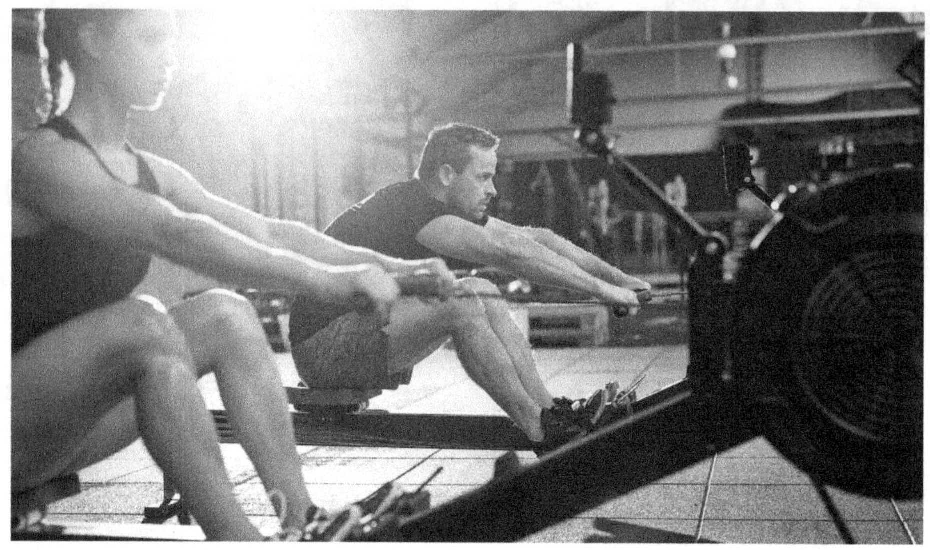

Core Strengthening Exercises

Maintaining proper alignment and posture is essential for keeping the body healthy and avoiding pain. Because they give the spine and pelvis stability and support, our core muscles are essential for this. Somatic exercises are an excellent way to strengthen your core, correct posture, and enhance your general well-being because they place a strong emphasis on internal awareness and gentle movement.

Advantages of Somatic Exercises for Strengthening the Core

Doing somatic core exercises regularly has various advantages:

1. Better alignment and posture are the result of stronger core muscles, which also lessen the chance of pain by stabilizing and supporting the spine.
2. Improved core stability: As you engage your core more frequently during everyday tasks, movement efficiency increases and injury risk decreases.
3. Improved flexibility: Somatic exercises, which incorporate gentle stretches to improve flexibility in the surrounding muscles and core, can help you achieve better posture and movement.
4. Reducing stress: By connecting with your body's reaction to stress, somatic awareness enables you to let go of tension and encourage relaxation.

Exercises for Somatic Core Strengthening

Here are three somatic core exercises that are easy to do anywhere and are very effective:

1. Dog Bird:

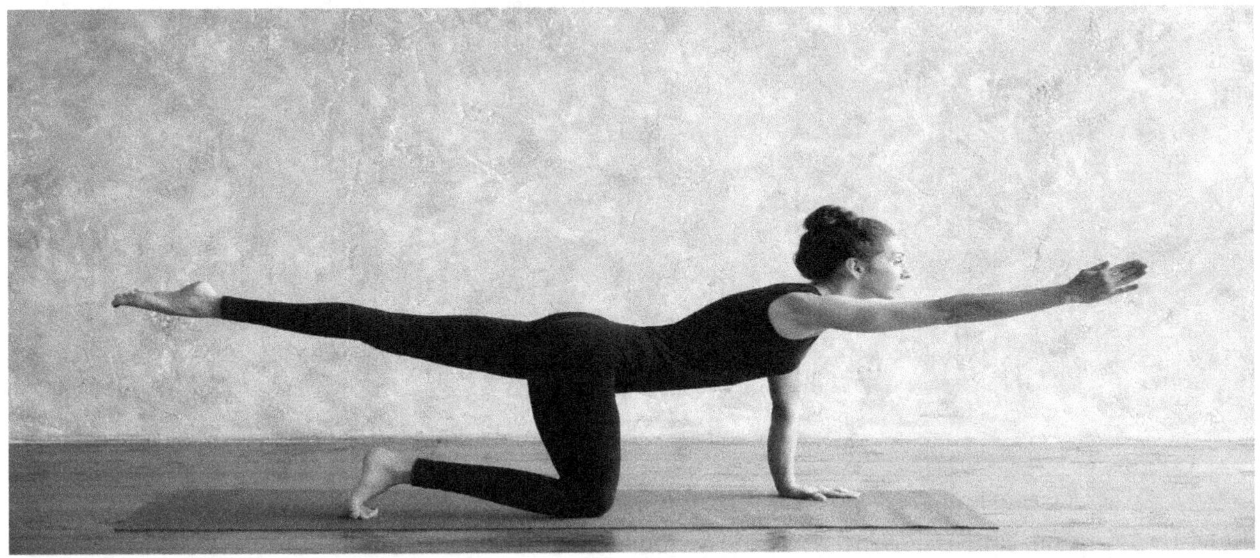

Maintain a neutral spine as you begin on your hands and knees.

Maintaining a flat back and an engaged core, extend one arm forward and the opposing leg back.

Hold for a few breaths, keeping your spine straight and your core active.

Continue on the opposite side.

Work out 5–10 times on each side.

2. Reach-equipped side plank:

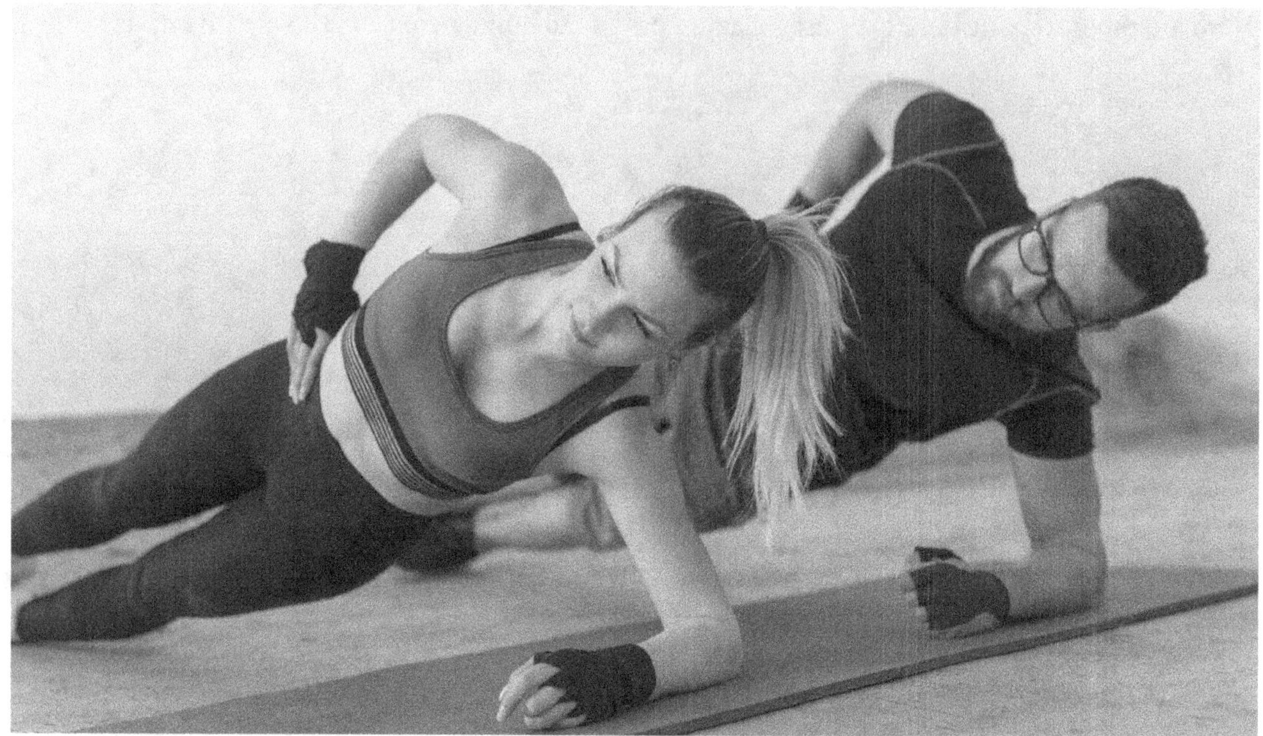

Start by lying on your side with your elbow bent to a 90-degree angle and your forearm directly under your shoulder.

Lift your body into a side plank position by stacking your hips and using your core.

Feel your side and core muscles contract as you extend your free arm overhead.

Hold while keeping your plank posture steady for a few breaths.

Continue on the opposite side.

Work out 5–10 times on each side.

3. Dead Bug

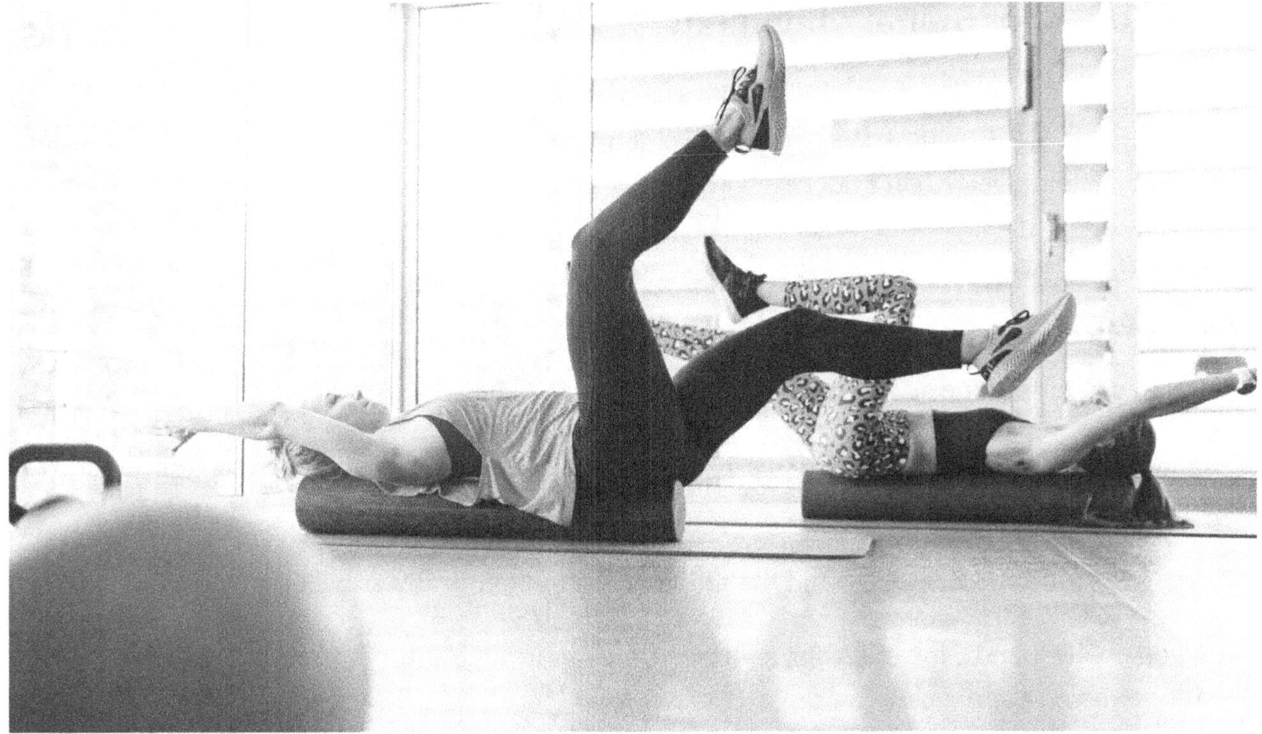

With your feet flat on the ground and your knees bent, lie on your back.

Engage your core and gently press your lower back into the floor.

As you slowly extend one arm and the opposing leg straight out, firmly support your lower back.

For a few breaths, hold the position while keeping your spine neutral and your core engaged.

Continue on the opposite side.

Work out 5–10 times on each side.

Extra Advice:

Take slow, deep breaths during each exercise.

Pay attention to your body and steer clear of any painful movements.

Rather than attempting to force movement, concentrate on using your core muscles correctly.

For best results, perform these exercises regularly.

Techniques for Spinal Alignment

Sustaining optimal spinal alignment is essential for mitigating pain and discomfort and augmenting general health. With somatic practices, you can cultivate awareness and release tension, which are gentle yet effective ways to improve your spinal alignment.

1. Cat-Cow with Awareness of Spine:

(page 26, fig.2)

Maintain a neutral spine as you begin on your hands and knees.

Take a deep breath and arch your back like a cat, emphasizing to lengthen your spine and lower your belly to the floor.

Sensate the stretch in your chest and the mild extension in your lower back.

Pull your belly button toward your spine and tuck your chin into your chest as you release the breath, rounding your back like a cow.

During this exercise, pay attention to your lower back's natural curve.

While you repeat this flow five to ten times, keep your awareness of your spinal movement.

2. Spinal Twist:

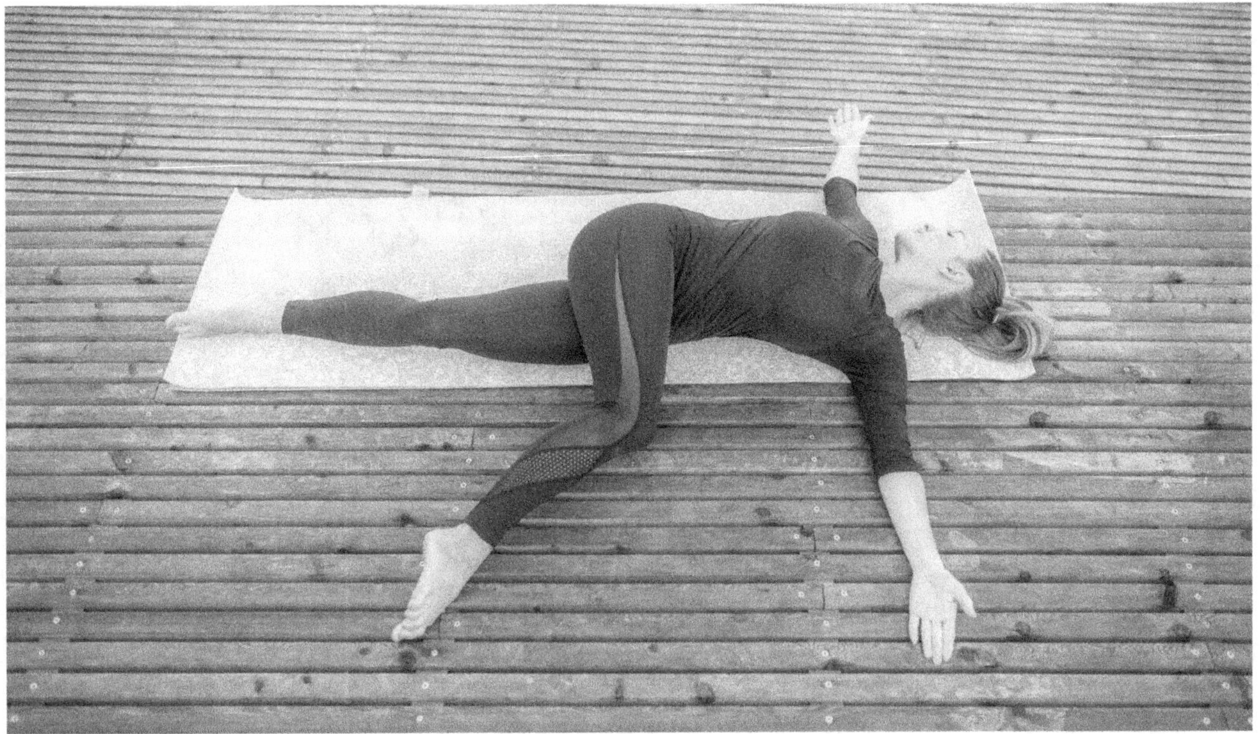

With your feet flat on the ground and your knees bent, lie comfortably on your back.

For support, place a rolled towel or bolster beneath your knees.

As much as is comfortable, sag your knees gently to one side and let your spine naturally twist.

Keep your shoulders back and firmly planted on the ground.

For a few breaths, hold this posture, concentrating on any sensations in your back and letting go of any tension.

Continue on the opposite side.

3. Rolls of the spine while standing:

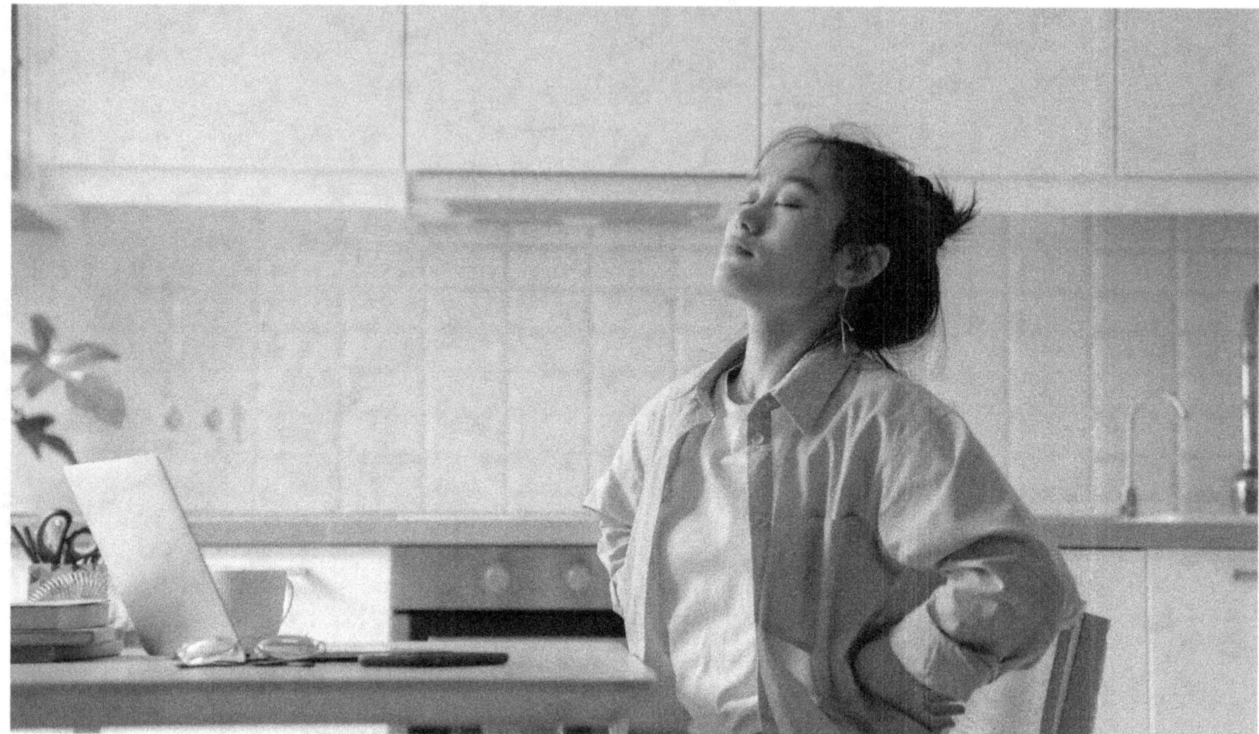

Place your feet hip-width apart and bend your knees just a little bit.

With your thumbs pointing back, place your hands on your lower back.

Start by gradually rolling your spine, vertebra by vertebra, starting at your tailbone and working your way up through your neck.

Roll forward 5-7 times, then reverse direction and roll backward for the same number of repetitions.

Continue breathing steadily, and refrain from jerky or forced movements.

Extra Advice:

Take slow, deep breaths during each exercise.

Pay attention to your body and steer clear of any painful movements.

With a gentle awareness, concentrate on releasing tension and mobilizing your spine.

For best results, perform these exercises regularly.

Balance and Stability Training

Balance and stability are essential for daily activities and overall well-being. Somatic exercises can help refine your proprioception (bodily awareness) and strengthen your core muscles, leading to improved balance and stability.

1. Single-Leg Stand with Eyes Closed:

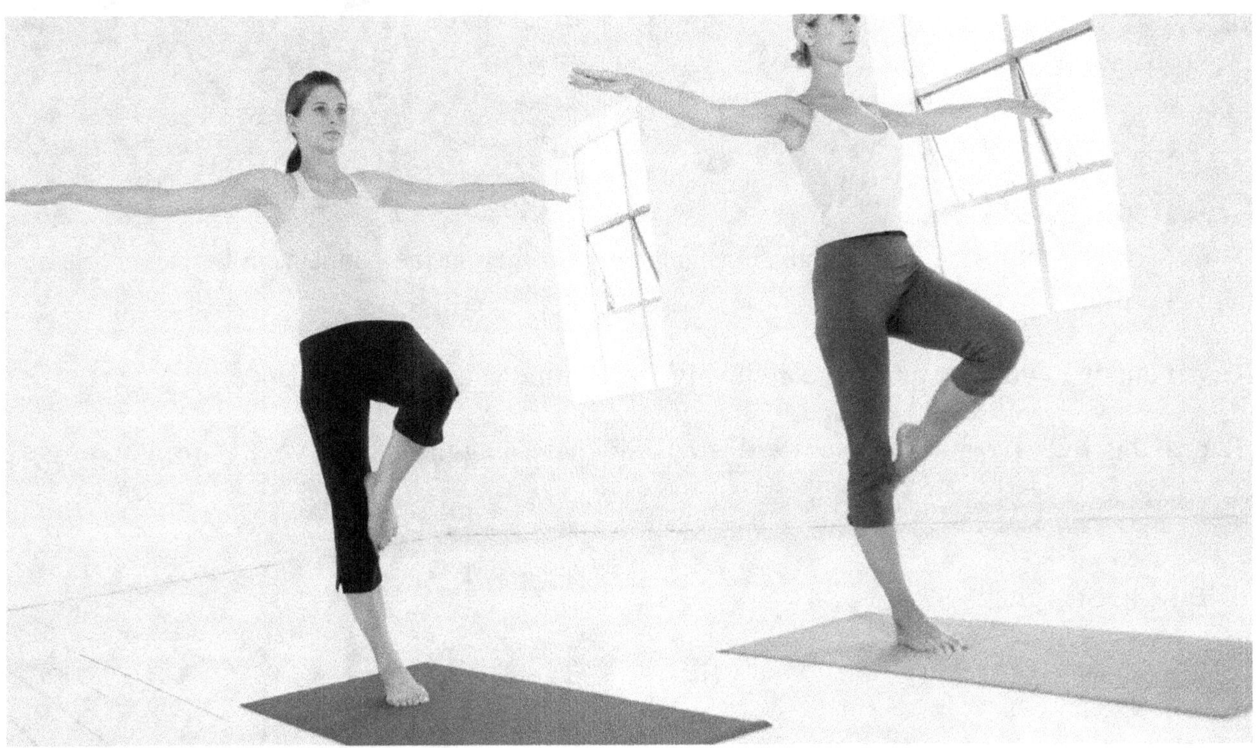

Stand with your feet hip-width apart and find a stable surface nearby for support if needed.

Slowly shift your weight onto one leg and softly lift the other foot off the ground, maintaining your hips level.

Close your eyes and hold for 5-10 seconds, focusing on balancing and maintaining a strong core engagement.

Continue on the opposite side.

Gradually increase the holding time as you improve.

2. Heel-Toe Walk:

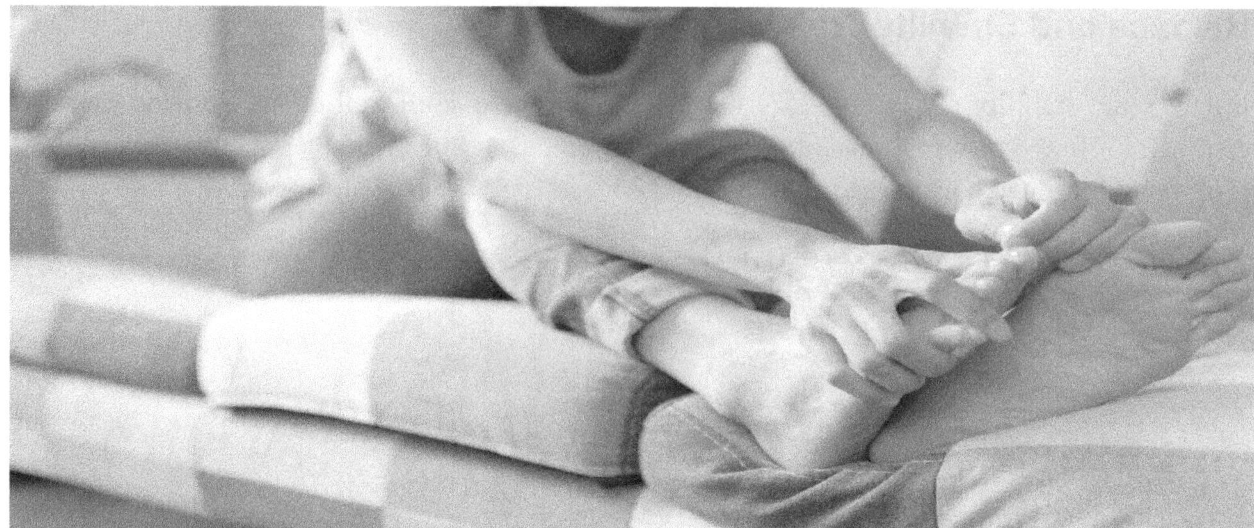

Walk slowly heel-to-toe in a straight line, focusing on feeling the connection between your feet and the earth.

Pay attention to your posture and core involvement while you maintain balance.

Repeat this walk forward and backward, gradually increasing the pace as your control improves.

3. Tai Chi Stepping:

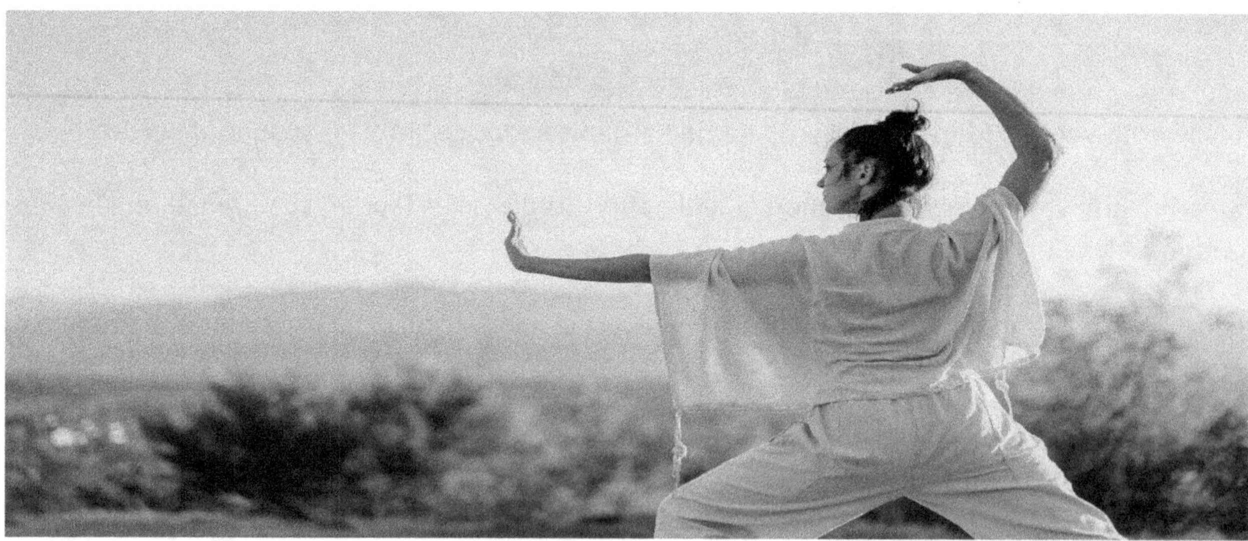

Stand with your feet slightly wider than shoulder-width apart and knees slightly bent.

Shift your weight to one leg and slowly extend the other leg forward, keeping your heel flat on the ground.

Sink your hips slightly as you extend your leg and feel your core engage for stability.

Gently lift your back leg forward and repeat the step with the other leg.

Focus on conscious movement and breathing as you flow through the stepping pattern.

Extra Advice:

Start with modest movements and gradually raise the challenge as you develop confidence.

Pay attention to your posture and core involvement throughout the workouts.

Practice regularly to enhance your balance and stability over time.

Consistency is crucial! By adding these somatic techniques into your everyday routine, you can enjoy improved spinal alignment, better balance, and enhanced general well-being.

CHAPTER SIX

ENHANCING FLEXIBILITY AND RANGE OF MOTION

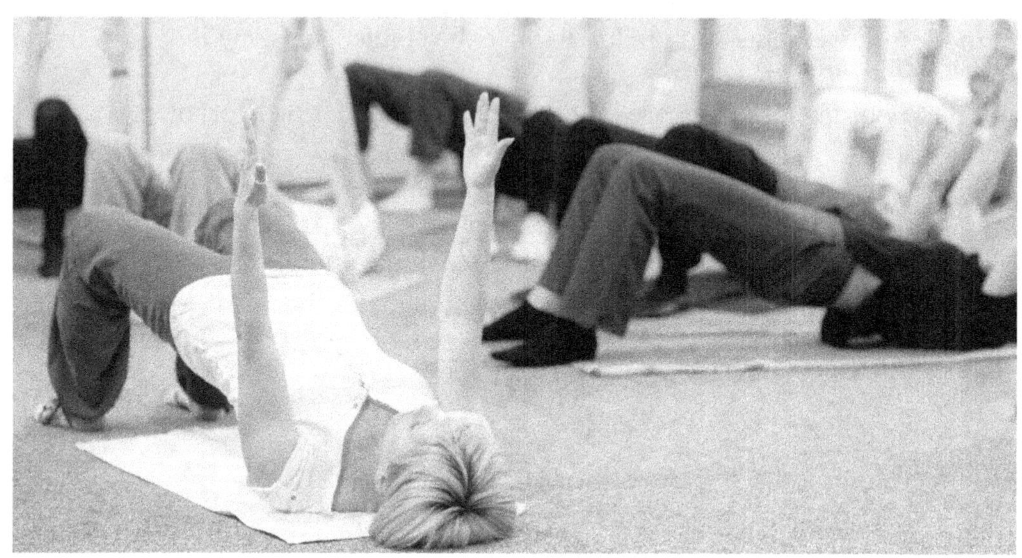

Joint Mobilization Techniques

Enhancing flexibility and range of motion adds to better strength, injury prevention, and total physical freedom. Somatic exercises, with their emphasis on gentle movement and internal awareness, offer efficient joint mobilization approaches to attain this goal.

Benefits of Somatic Joint Mobilization:

1. Regular practice of somatic joint mobilization gives various benefits:
2. Increased flexibility and range of motion: Gentle mobilization reduces tightness and increases movement in your joints, making everyday activities easier and more comfortable.
3. Reduced pain and stiffness: Mobilizing joints helps alleviate stiffness and discomfort, boosting overall well-being.
4. Better joint health: Mild exercise helps to maintain the long-term health of your joints by lubricating and feeding them.
5. Enhanced body awareness: During mobilization, paying attention to internal feelings strengthens your bond with your body and its requirements.

Methods of Somatic Joint Mobilization:

Here are three easy-to-use yet powerful methods you can try:

1. Gently Rotate Your Arms:

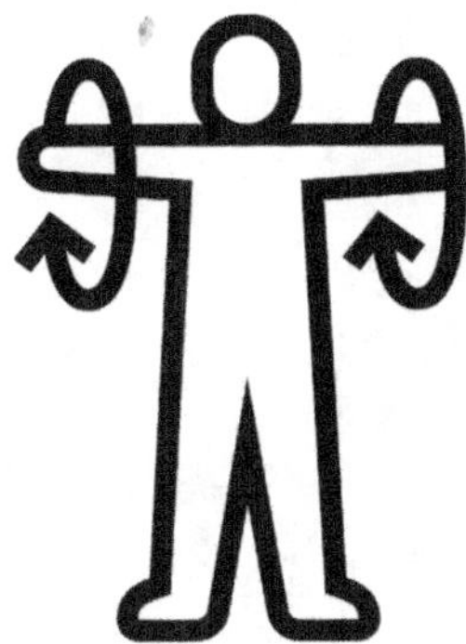

Maintain a relaxed stance with your feet hip-width apart.

Start by slowly tracing little circles with your arms, moving them forward and backward alternately.

Instead of making jerky movements, concentrate on sensing the movement inside your shoulder joints.

Increase the circle's size gradually as your range of motion permits.

In each direction, repeat five to ten circles.

2. Bending the knee while rotating:

Place your feet hip-width apart and bend your knees just a little bit.

Start bending your knees gradually while paying attention to how your knee joints move.

One at a time, slowly rotate your knees inward and then outward as you approach the bottom of the bend.

Without attempting to move, feel the stretch in the muscles and tissues around you.

On each side, perform five to ten bends while rotating.

3. Twists in the spine:

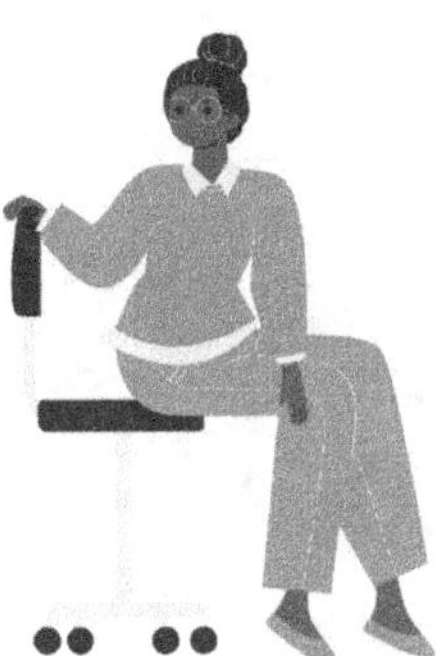

With your legs folded and your back straight, take a seat on a chair or the ground.

Feel the rotation in your muscles and spine as you slowly rotate your upper body to one side.

To prevent straining your neck, keep your hips looking forward.

After a few breaths of holding, move back to the middle and repeat on the opposite side.

Twist five to ten times on each side.

Extra Advice:

- Take slow, deep breaths during each workout.
- Pay attention to your body and steer clear of any painful motions.
- Concentrate on letting go of stress and flexing your joints softly.
- For best outcomes, put these strategies into regular practice.

Dynamic Stretching Sequences

Although flexibility has historically been linked to static stretching, somatic activities provide a dynamic approach by simulating ordinary motions through sequences. These exercises emphasize slow, deliberate movements and mild activation, which primes your body for action and expands its range of motion.

Advantages of Sequences with Dynamic Stretching:

1. Better muscle activation: Dynamic stretches work your muscles by using deliberate motions that increase their reactivity and coordination.
2. Lower chance of injury: Stretching statically increases the danger of strains and tears in your muscles. Preparing your muscles for exercise helps avoid these injuries.
3. Improved coordination and agility: Moving through dynamic sequences makes it easier for your body to move effectively and fluidly.
4. Heart rate and blood flow are raised: These movements work as a mild warm-up, raising your heart rate and getting your body ready for exercise.

Example of a Dynamic Stretching Sequence

This sequence is merely an example. Think about customizing it to your requirements and degree of fitness.

1. Arm circles: Start small and work your way up to larger forward and backward circles.
2. Arm swings: As you swing your arms back and forth, notice how your shoulders and upper back become active.
3. Torso twists: While maintaining your hips pointing forward, gently rotate your torso back and forth.
4. Leg swings: With a controlled motion and an engaged core, swing each leg forward and backward.
5. High knees: While running, raise your knees to your chest while staying in position.
6. Lunges with arm reaches: Take a step forward and raise your opposing arm above your head. Continue on the opposite side.
7. Jumping jacks: Execute this exercise by making deliberate leaps and landing gently.

Extra Advice:

Breathe easily and deeply the entire way through the sequence.

Avoid ballistic motions and concentrate on calm ones.

When necessary, modify the intensity based on your body's feedback.

Include this sequence in your warm-up before doing any exercises or activities requiring a lot of flexibility.

Whole-Body Flexibility Exercises:

Somatic full-body exercises combine mobilizations, conscious transitions, and mild stretches to improve flexibility from all angles. These exercises increase your range of motion throughout your entire body, reduce tension, and foster body awareness.

Advantages of Whole-Body Flexibility Exercises

1. Enhanced flexibility throughout the body: By focusing on the main joints and muscle groups, these exercises help you become more flexible all over.
2. Better alignment and posture: Better flexibility naturally results in better alignment and posture, which lessens discomfort and potential pain.
3. Stress reduction: These routines' mindfulness component relieves tension and encourages mental and physical relaxation.
4. Better physical health: Increased flexibility helps with everyday tasks, athletic performance, and general physical health.

Full-Body Flexibility Routine:

This method is merely an example. You are welcome to change it to suit your needs and tastes.

Shoulders and neck: Start with light shrugs, shoulder circles, and neck rolls.

Spine: Do side bends, supported spinal twists, and cat-cow poses.

Include lunges, figure-four stretches, and light hip circles for your legs and hips.

Stretches for the hamstrings and glutes should be combined with downward-facing dog and supported forward folds.

Back and chest: Work on arm circles, mild back arches, and supported chest openers.

Extra Advice:

- Take slow, deep breaths during each workout.
- Let go of any tension and concentrate on the feelings in your body.
- With slow breaths, hold each stretch for 20 to 30 seconds.
- For best effects, repeat the process two to three times a week.

CHAPTER SEVEN

SOMATIC EXERCISES FOR STRESSFUL SITUATIONS

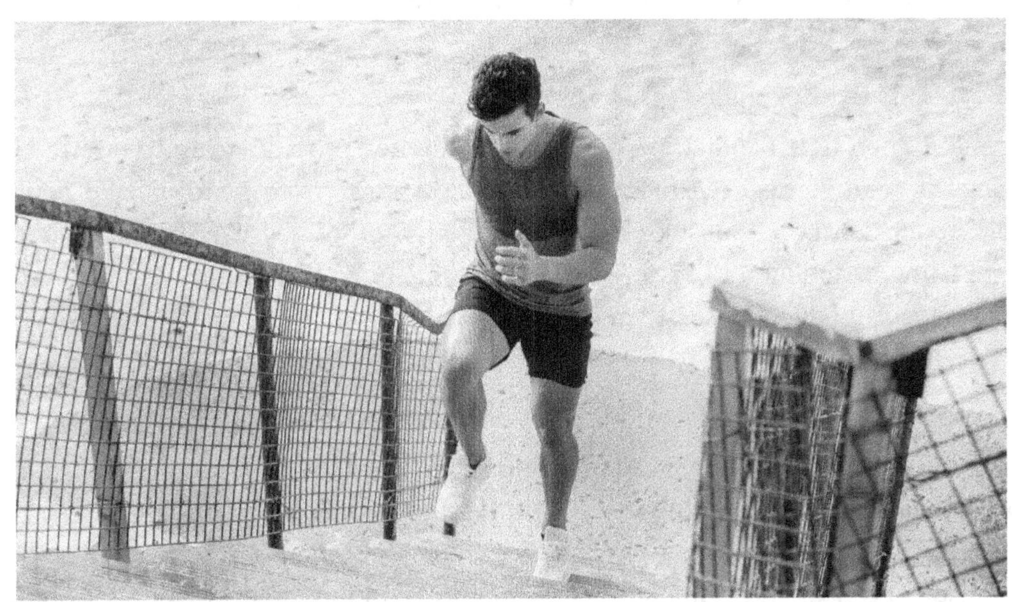

Including somatic techniques can provide a haven of resilience and serenity in the face of difficult circumstances, amidst the everyday chaos. Here, we explore particular somatic practices intended to encourage calmness, lessen tension, and reestablish equilibrium during trying times:

Stressful circumstances can set off a chain reaction of physical and mental reactions, but with somatic exercises, people can develop a sense of centering and tranquility that promotes resilience and overall well-being. A closer look at useful somatic exercises designed for high-stress scenarios is provided below:

1. Conscious Breathing:

When people are under stress, mindful breathing acts as a strong anchor that enables them to control their mental and physical reactions. By focusing on the sensations of the breath as it enters and exits the body, such as the rise and fall of the abdomen or the sensation of air going through the nose, people can engage in mindful breathing. People who breathe deeply and rhythmically trigger a relaxation response in their bodies, which helps them feel stable and at ease even in the middle of chaos.

2. Grounding Methods:

By establishing a connection with one's body and surroundings, one can anchor oneself in the present moment through the use of grounding practices. One easy grounding technique is to focus on the feelings of stability and support that come from your feet as they make contact with the earth. People can also walk mindfully to practice grounding, paying attention to their movements and the feelings they feel in their bodies with each stride.

3. Practices of Somatic Movement:

During stressful conditions, somatic movement techniques provide a mild yet effective way to induce relaxation and release tension. One somatic exercise is to gently shake or tremble the body to release tension in the muscles and allow energy to flow freely. Slow, conscious motions like soft stretching, reaching, or twisting are another technique that promotes the development of embodied presence and the release of tension.

4. PMR, or progressive muscle relaxation, is:

Tensing and relaxing particular muscle regions to encourage profound relaxation is the methodical relaxation technique known as Progressive Muscle Relaxation (PMR). People can practice progressive muscle relaxation (PMR) in stressful situations by gradually tensing and releasing muscle groups, beginning at the feet and working their way up the body. People encourage relaxation and lessen the physiological impacts of stress by releasing tense muscles.

5. Guided imagery and visualization:

In the middle of chaos, visualization and guided imagery provide a haven of peace. People can engage in visualization exercises by visualizing themselves in a calm and quiet setting, such as a lush forest or a pleasant beach. Another useful tool for encouraging relaxation and stress reduction is guided imagery scripts or recordings, which can take users through peaceful sceneries or scenarios.

6. Inhalation-Based Movement:

Breath-centric movement techniques combine mindful breathing with soft movement to encourage the body's natural flow and relaxation. One such is mindful walking, in which participants coordinate their breathing with each stride to develop a sense of rhythm and present-moment awareness. Another technique that promotes embodiment and relaxation is light yoga or tai chi motions timed with the breath.

Somatic exercises provide a toolkit of techniques for handling stressful circumstances with composure and strength. People can develop a sense of peace and center by integrating breath-centric movement, progressive muscle relaxation, somatic movement practices, grounding techniques, visualization, and mindful breathing into their daily lives. This will promote health and vitality even in the face of life's obstacles.

Relief from Desk Work

Extended periods spent seated at a desk can cause both physical and mental exhaustion. Desk-bound alleviation techniques provide simple, efficient means of reducing stress and reviving energy:

1. Spinal Twist on a Chair:

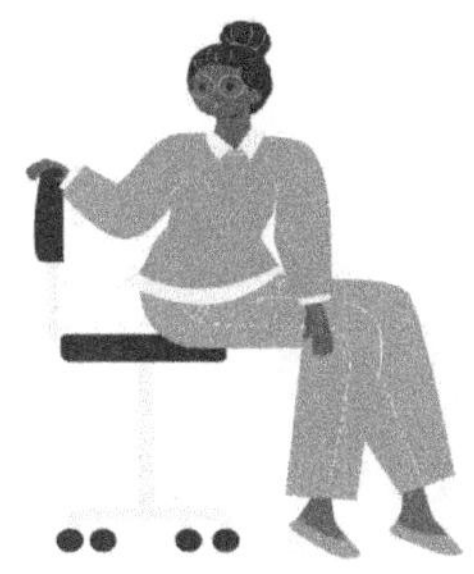

With one hand on the knee across from you and the other on the chair's back, slowly rotate your torso to one side while seated. Repeat on the opposite side after holding the twist for a few breaths. This easy motion enhances mobility and relieves tension in the spine.

2. **Rolls of the shoulders:**

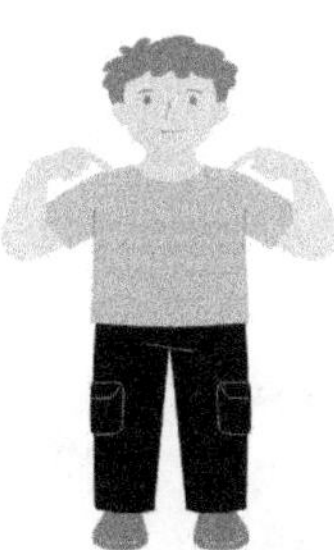

Raise your shoulders to your ears, then slowly roll them back and forth in a circle. Repeat multiple times, letting your movements be deliberate and slow. Shoulder rolls facilitate relaxation and lessen stiffness by releasing tension in the neck and shoulders.

3. Hand and Wrist Extensions:

With your palm facing down, extend one arm in front of you. Using your other hand, gently grip the fingers and draw them back towards you until your wrist and forearm start to stretch. After a few breaths of holding, switch sides. This stretch relieves the strain from extended mouse or keyboard use.

4. Folding a desk forward:

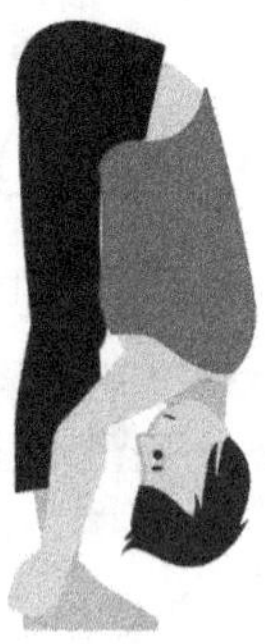

Sitting, push your chair back a little and bend forward at the hips so that your upper body folds over your lower thighs. Breathe deeply for a while while placing your forehead on your arms or the surface of your desk. This soft forward fold facilitates relaxation by releasing tension in the shoulders and back.

Comfortable Transportation

Walking, taking public transportation, or driving a car daily can all be demanding and exhausting. Including somatic exercises in your commute can ease pain and encourage relaxation:

1. Conscious Breathing:

Spend some time concentrating on your breathing during your commute. Breathe deeply through your nose, expanding your abdomen, and then slowly release any tension or stress by exhaling through your mouth. To induce relaxation and soothe the nervous system, mindful breathing is helpful.

2. Shoulder and neck rolls:

When sitting at a stop sign or on public transit, gently roll your shoulders and neck to relieve tension. Roll your shoulders forward and backward after slowly rotating your head from side to side. This easy exercise facilitates mobility and relieves tightness in the shoulders and neck.

3. Cat-Cow Stretch in Sitting:

Use a seated variation of the cat-cow stretch if you're riding a seat. Place your hands on your knees and sit up straight. Breathe in as you raise your chest and arch your back (cow), and release as you bend your back and tuck your chin in toward your chest (cat). To improve posture and relieve tension in the spine, repeat multiple times.

4. Concise Observation:

Make the most of your commute by taking the time to carefully observe your surroundings. Observe the sights, sounds, and feelings in your immediate environment without bias or connection. This present-moment awareness technique can ease tension and foster a feeling of peace and connectedness.

These specific somatic exercises can help you decompress, encourage relaxation, and improve your general well-being in the face of modern life's pressures. You can incorporate them into your daily commute and workstation routine.

Relaxing Methods for Busy Days

Finding quiet times during hectic days can seem like a luxury. Quick and efficient relaxing methods, however, can drastically lower stress levels, sharpen focus, and improve general well-being when included in a daily routine. Here are some somatically based techniques to help you find calm in the middle of the chaos:

1. Five-Minute Body Scan:

Locate a peaceful area and take a comfortable seat or lie down.

Shut your eyes and concentrate on your breathing while noticing the rise and fall in your abdomen.

Focus on your toes and slowly scan your upper body, taking note of any feelings without passing judgment.

With every breath out, notice any tightness or tension and visualize releasing it.

Keep looking around your body, paying particular attention to your chest, neck, and head as well as your main muscle groups.

As you get to your head, picture a calm, still feeling enveloping your entire body.

Open your eyes gradually and retain this serene sensation as you do so.

2. Observant Breath:

With your shoulders relaxed and your back upright, take a comfortable seat.

If you would like, soften your sight or close your eyes.

Pay attention to your breathing and the sensation of air entering and exiting your nose.

Silently count to ten before taking another breath.

Bring your focus back to your breathing softly and without passing judgment if your thoughts stray.

For three to five minutes, practice this, letting your breath serve as your anchor in the here and now.

3. Progressive Relaxation of the Muscles:

Shut your eyes while you comfortably sit or lie down.

Gradually tense and release different muscle groups, working your way up your body from your toes.

For instance, grip your toes tightly for a short while, then relax by releasing them.

Repeat this for your face, neck, arms, legs, buttocks, abdominal muscles, chest, and back.

Imagine the stress leaving your body as you release each muscle group and being replaced by a profound state of relaxation.

4. Assisted Visualization:

Locate a peaceful area and settle in.

Shut your eyes and picture yourself in a tranquil, serene setting.

This might be any place that inspires sentiments of calm and quiet, such as a beach, forest, or garden.

Activate your senses by visualizing the sights, sounds, textures, and scents of your tranquil space.

Give this visualization your complete attention and feel the serenity pour into your body and mind.

Take a few minutes to remain in this tranquil condition, and then slowly make your way back to your surroundings.

5. Brief Interval of Movement:

Take a few deep breaths and stand up.

Bend from side to side, extend your arms overhead, and gently roll your shoulders.

Spend a few minutes strolling around while paying attention to your body's motions and the feelings in your feet.

This brief period of activity can help you decompress and revitalize.

Extra Advice:

Regularly put these strategies into practice, even when you're not experiencing stress.

As you get more comfortable, gradually extend the time from the shorter starting points.

These methods can be combined with additional self-care routines such as writing, going for walks outdoors, or listening to relaxing music.

Recall that even brief mindfulness exercises can have a significant impact on stress reduction and well-being enhancement.

CHAPTER EIGHT

ESTABLISHING YOUR SOMATIC ROUTINE

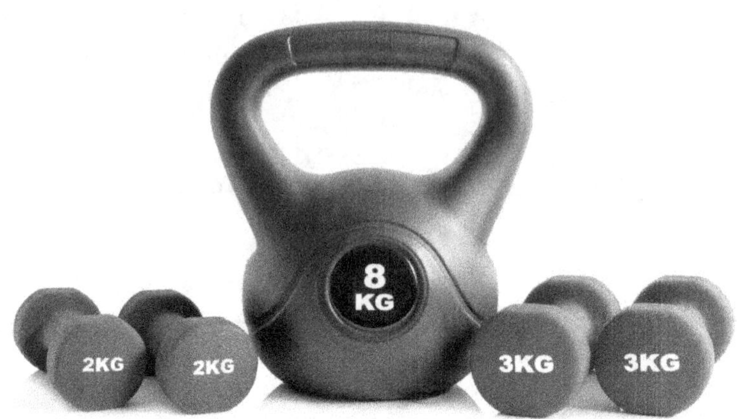

Setting aspirations is the first step in developing your somatic routine. Your somatic practice takes on a specific trajectory based on your intentions, which work as guiding principles to match your activities with your goals and wishes. This article examines the importance of intention-setting and offers helpful advice on how to incorporate this essential step into your daily routine:

Developing a personal somatic practice enables you to develop self-awareness, improve health, and promote overall development. Here, we explore the fundamental action of intention-setting and how it can completely change your somatic journey:

Defining Goals:

Establishing intentions for your somatic practice entails defining your goals and developing a concentrated mentality. Whether your goals are to achieve emotional equilibrium, physical well-being, stress reduction, or relaxation, intentions serve as a compass that directs your actions. Setting goals is essential while developing your somatic regimen for the following reasons:

1. Direction and Defining Terms: Your goals for your somatic practice can be identified with the use of intentions, which provide direction and clarity. By stating your intentions clearly, you

build a road map that guides you in choosing methods, exercises, and routines that support your objectives.

2. Compliance with Principles: You can harmonize your somatic practice with your fundamental beliefs and values by setting intentions. You may customize your somatic routine to honor these values and support holistic well-being by thinking about what's most important to you. This could be developing resilience, self-compassion, or self-care.

3. Drive and Dedication: Your dedication to your somatic practice is fueled by your intentions, which are strong motivators. You can develop a sense of purpose and dedication that keeps you involved over time, even in the face of obstacles or disappointments, by clearly and firmly stating your aims.

4. Concentration and Awareness: By establishing goals, you can improve mindfulness in your somatic practice and develop a focused mentality. You can cultivate more self-awareness and embodiment by staying present and involved in every minute of your practice by focusing your attention on your aims.

5. Flexibility and Adaptability: With intentions, you have a framework that is flexible enough to respond and adjust to your changing requirements and circumstances. By refining and adjusting your intents as you move through your somatic journey, you can make sure that your practice stays dynamic and receptive to your growth, even if your goals, priorities, and experiences change.

Useful Advice for Setting Intentions

1. Consider Your Why: Give some thought to the reasons behind your attraction to somatic activities and the outcomes you intend to achieve. Think about the areas of your life where you want to be more aligned or transformed, and then choose intents that support these goals.

2. Write Them Down: Express your goals in writing using language that speaks to you in a clear, affirming manner. Put them on paper in a diary, make a vision board, or put them somewhere noticeable so you can see them often to serve as a reminder and source of inspiration.

3. Cultivate Presence: As you make your intentions, practice mindfulness and presence to enable a profound connection with your inner guidance and intuition. When creating

intentions that seem real and significant to you, follow your heart's desires and have faith in your instincts.

4. Remain Open and Curious: As you delve into many facets of your somatic practice, keep an open mind and a curious spirit. Accept exploration and learning, letting your goals develop naturally as you become more deeply involved with somatic methods and practices.

Establishing clear, motivating, and goal- and value-aligned intents is the first step towards developing your somatic practice. By developing intentionality and mindfulness in your somatic practice, you give yourself the ability to set out on a life-changing path of self-awareness, development, and well-being.

Designing Your Practice Space

The quality of your somatic experience is greatly influenced by the design of your practice area, which creates an environment that is conducive to embodiment, relaxation, and focus. How to create a room that facilitates your somatic practice is as follows:

1. Clutter-Free Ambience: Establish a clutter-free atmosphere that encourages roominess and peace. To foster a sense of peace and tranquility, clear your practice area of extraneous distractions and clutter.

2. Comfortable Flooring or Seating: Select flooring or seating that allows you to sit comfortably and maintain an upright, relaxed posture. Whether it's a comfortable blanket, a chair with support, or a cushioned mat, make sure your seating arrangement promotes comfort and mobility.

3. Natural Light and Ventilation: To create a bright and airy atmosphere, maximize the amount of natural light and ventilation in your practice area. To improve the atmosphere, add soft lighting alternatives like candles or dimmable lamps or open the windows to let in natural sunlight and fresh air.

4. Personal Touches: Add unique elements to your practice area that express your beliefs, interests, and preferences. Embrace things that inspire and provide comfort, whether it's somber colors, sentimental artifacts, or works of art that inspire you.

5. Organizational mechanisms: Put in place organizational mechanisms to maintain a clean and functional practice area. For easy access and neat organization of props, accessories, and equipment, use storage solutions like baskets, shelves, or drawers.

Achieving Uniformity

In somatic practices, consistency is the cornerstone of growth and advancement, encouraging perseverance, discipline, and journey continuation. Here's how to make your somatic practice consistent:

1. Set Achievable Goals: Considering your priorities, schedule, and commitments, set attainable goals for your somatic practice. Divide more ambitious objectives into more doable milestones, and design a disciplined schedule that accommodates frequent practice sessions.

2. Establish a Routine: Make sure your somatic practice is consistent by blocking out specific times on your daily or weekly calendar for practice sessions. Consider your somatic practice to

be an appointment with oneself that cannot be changed; give it the same priority as any other significant commitment.

3. Start Tiny and Develop Momentum: As you gain confidence and momentum, progressively extend the length and intensity of your practice sessions. Begin with tiny, reasonable time increments. Focus on attending regularly, even if it's only for a little while each day, as consistency is more significant than duration.

4. Locate Accountability Partners: Look for communities or accountability partners who are interested in somatic practices and who can offer accountability, support, and encouragement. Become a member of local communities, social media platforms, or online forums to meet like-minded people and discuss your achievements and difficulties.

5. Monitor Your Progress: Keep a practice notebook or log to record your advancements and successes in your somatic practice. Keep a journal of your observations, learnings, and experiences, documenting any advancements or modifications to your mental, emotional, and physical health throughout time.

Creating a consistent practice environment and creating a supportive design are critical components in maximizing the efficacy of somatic practices. On your somatic journey, you lay the groundwork for significant transformation, growth, and well-being by establishing a loving environment and making a commitment to frequent practice.

CHAPTER NINE

BEYOND THE BASICS: EXPLORING ADVANCED SOMATIC PRACTICES

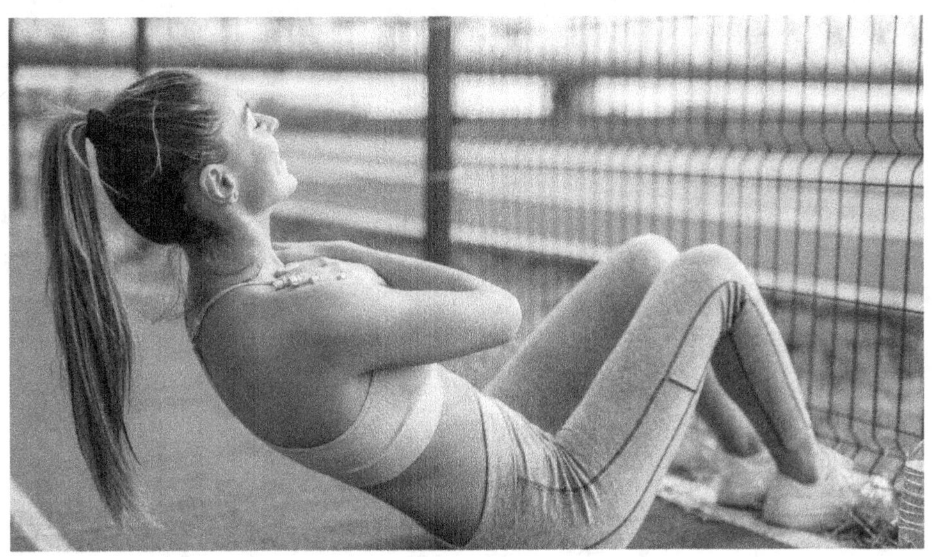

Exploring advanced practices becomes a logical next step as your somatic journey develops, leading to deeper comprehension and embodiment. Movement integration exercises combine movement, self-awareness, and mindfulness in a transformative way, providing a sophisticated method of somatic exploration. This article explores movement integration exercises as a means of improving embodiment and achieving holistic well-being. It delves into the field of advanced somatic practices.

Beyond the fundamentals of somatic techniques, one can access profound depths of embodiment, transformation, and self-discovery. Here, using movement integration activities, we delve into the more complex area of somatic exploration:

Exercises for Movement Integration

Movement integration exercises offer a dynamic approach to embodied discovery and self-expression by fusing conscious movement with somatic concepts. An in-depth examination of movement integration exercises and their potential for transformation is provided below:

1. Movement Integration Principles: Somatic awareness, mindfulness, and movement exploration serve as the foundation for movement integration exercises. These exercises focus on the integration of the mind, body, and spirit by encouraging self-awareness, presence, and vitality through deliberate movement activities.

2. Mindful Movement Sequences: Mindful movement sequences are a type of movement integration exercise that focuses on using the entire body in a fluid, expressive, and deliberate manner. Dynamic exercises like tai chi forms, flowing yoga sequences, or somatic movement explorations that encourage people to move mindfully and intentionally could be included in these sequences.

3. Embodied Exploration: By encouraging embodied investigation of movement patterns, feelings, and emotions, movement integration exercises help people develop a better comprehension of the relationship between the body and mind. With inquiry and openness, participants are urged to investigate movement variations, transitions, and qualities, tuning into subtle sensations and nuances of embodiment.

4. Somatic Inquiry and contemplation: Two fundamental elements of movement integration exercises are somatic inquiry and contemplation. Inquiring about their experiences with movement, identifying points of tension, resistance, or limitation, and investigating strategies to foster more ease, fluidity, and integration in their movement patterns are all encouraged for participants.

5. Creative Expression and Playfulness: Somatic inquiry incorporates creativity and playfulness through movement integration exercises. To foster a sense of freedom, joy, and self-expression via movement, participants are encouraged to try out movement improvisation, creative expression, and unplanned play.

6. Integration with Daily Life: Movement integration exercises cover interactions and activities that occur in daily life in addition to structured practice sessions. It is recommended that participants incorporate the ideas of mindful movement into their everyday routines. Some examples of this include walking attentively, moving mindfully while performing daily duties, and scheduling movement breaks during periods of inactivity.

To sum up, movement integration exercises invite participants to enhance their embodiment, self-awareness, and connection to the present moment through a comprehensive approach to somatic inquiry. On their advanced somatic journey, individuals can unleash new depths of energy, creativity, and well-being by practicing mindful movement that integrates the body, mind, and spirit.

Somatic Investigation Using Yoga or Dance

Yoga and dance are two exquisite mediums for somatic inquiry, each providing special interior journeys through movement. Which one you choose will rely on your tastes and aspirations:

Dance: Expressive movement: Dancing promotes instinctive, unrestricted movement that enables you to become aware of the feelings in your body and let them out via expressive movements.

fun and creativity: The emphasis is on discovery and the enjoyment of movement, encouraging fun and individual expression.

Diversity of styles: Different dance genres, such as ballet, improvisation, and modern, are available to suit diverse requirements and tastes.

Yoga: Mindfulness and Breathwork: This form of exercise focuses on deliberate movement and mindful breathing to promote introspection and mental calmness.

Structured poses: Asanas, or poses, work on particular energy pathways and muscle groups to increase awareness and flexibility.

Range of methods: Diverse yoga styles, ranging from soothing Hatha to energetic Vinyasa, accommodate a range of fitness levels and objectives.

Selecting the Appropriate Course:
1. Contemplation: Do you like structured guidance and contemplation, or do you seek independence and the ability to express yourself via movement?
2. Physicality: Take into account your degree of fitness and any physical restrictions. Although forms of yoga and dance differ in intensity, they both provide adaptations.
3. Personal preference: Try out several instructors and programs to see what feels right for you on an emotional and physical level.

Cooperating with Practitioners of Somatics

Your path of somatic discovery can be greatly aided by somatic practitioners. How they can help you is as follows:
1. Personalized guidance: They evaluate your requirements and design procedures that are specific to your goals and body.
2. Education on movement: They assist you in comprehending your movement patterns and pinpointing areas that require development.

3. Injury prevention: They help you move properly and prevent injuries; they are especially helpful for people who already have medical concerns.
4. Emotional release: Some instructors incorporate movement with emotional inquiry to assist you in expressing and letting go of pent-up feelings.
5. Locating a Professional:
6. Qualifications: Seek out licensed dance movement therapists, somatic movement educators, or bodywork therapists.
7. Specialization: Certain practitioners focus on particular fields, such as movement disorders, trauma healing, or pain treatment.
8. Consultation: Arrange a meeting to talk about your objectives and make sure we're a good fit.

Extra Advice:

1. Begin cautiously: Start with one or two sessions a week and work your way up depending on your needs.
2. Open communication: Let your practitioner know if you are uncomfortable or have any questions.
3. Self-practice: To enhance your sessions, include self-guided somatic activities in your regimen.

Remember that there is no one "correct" technique to investigate somatic practices. Through movement and awareness, you can start a personalized journey of self-discovery and well-being through yoga, dance, and working with practitioners.

CONCLUSION

Choosing to follow the road of somatic wellness is a life-changing adventure rather than just a trip. As we come to the end of our investigation into the field of somatic practices, it is clear that somatic wellness is a holistic way of life that integrates the body, mind, and spirit in harmonious interdependence. It goes beyond simple physical exercise or relaxation methods.

We have explored the fundamental ideas of somatics throughout this journey, realizing the close relationship between the mind and body and how somatic practices can be a doorway to improved well-being. We've seen firsthand how somatic activities may foster presence, resilience, and vitality in everything from mild movement explorations to complex integration exercises.

The call to embody presence—to become aware of the depth of our sensory experiences, to pay close attention to the guidance of our bodies, and to develop a strong sense of connection with both the outside world and ourselves—lays the foundation of somatic wellbeing. We can regain our intrinsic ability to heal, discover, and transform ourselves through somatic practices.

Let us approach somatic well-being with openness, curiosity, and compassion as we accept it as a lifelong path. Let's respect the knowledge that comes from our bodies and have faith in the inner intellect that directs us toward integration and wholeness. And let us never forget that every second, every breath, is a chance to return home to ourselves, to live fully alive, present, and joyfully.

Somatic wellbeing is a thread that runs through all facets of our lives, giving them significance, direction, and a sense of aliveness. May we keep walking this path with gratitude and humility, respecting the holiness of our bodies and bravely and gracefully embarking on the path to somatic wholeness?

We find a method of living as well as a way of being when we embrace somatic wellness, which is an invitation to dance with life in all its wonder, beauty, and complexity. We also discover liberty, embodiment, and the profound understanding that genuine well-being emerges from the depths of our physical presence in this dance.

Thus, let us go on this journey with open hearts and embodied minds, understanding that somatic wellness is a way of being—a means of welcoming life with vitality, authenticity, and love—rather than a destination. Accept the journey. Accept somatic health. Accept life as it is.

Glossary of Somatic Terms

1. Somatic: Relating to the body or bodily feelings; about the holistic integration of body, mind, and spirit.

2. Embodiment: The state of being fully present and aware in one's body; the integration of physical sensations, emotions, and thoughts into real experience.

3. Mind-Body Connection: The intricate relationship between mental and physical health, emphasizing the impact of ideas, emotions, and beliefs on bodily processes and vice versa.

4. Sensory Awareness: Conscious perception and recognition of bodily sensations, including touch, proprioception, and interoception, as a means of encouraging self-awareness and presence.

5. Breath Awareness: The practice of watching and regulating the breath to encourage relaxation, mindfulness, and physiological balance; a cornerstone of somatic practices.

6. Muscle Tension Release: Techniques aimed at releasing muscle tension and promoting relaxation, such as Progressive Muscle Relaxation (PMR) and myofascial release.

7. Movement Exploration: Deliberate and mindful exploration of movement patterns, ranges of motion, and physical capabilities as a means of promoting embodiment, mobility, and self-discovery.

8. Body Scan: A mindfulness exercise involving systematic attention to different regions of the body, often used to develop relaxation, awareness, and presence.

9. Grounding: Techniques for anchoring oneself in the present moment and creating a sense of stability and connection with the environment, often involving attention to the sensations of the body contacting the ground.

10. Somatic Exercises: Practices aimed at improving bodily awareness, movement efficiency, and overall well-being through mindful movement, breathwork, and self-awareness techniques.

11. Mindful Movement: Movement practices performed with conscious attention, purpose, and presence, emphasizing the integration of breath, movement, and awareness.

12. Integration: The process of assimilating and harmonizing various parts of experience, including physical sensations, emotions, thoughts, and behaviors, into a cohesive whole.

13. Presence: The state of being fully attentive, engaged, and aware in the present moment, embodying a feeling of openness, curiosity, and nonjudgmental awareness.

14. Resilience: The ability to adapt, recover, and thrive in the face of adversity, drawing upon inner resources, coping strategies, and supportive relationships.

15. Well-being: A holistic state of health and vitality encompassing physical, mental, emotional, and spiritual aspects, characterized by a sense of balance, fulfillment, and flourishing.

WORKOUT PLANNER

Workout PLANNER

Week _______________________ Month _______________________

	WORKOUT	MEALS	GOALS
Monday			

	WORKOUT	MEALS	GOALS
Tuesday			

	WORKOUT	MEALS	GOALS
Wednesday			

	WORKOUT	MEALS	GOALS
Thursday			

	WORKOUT	MEALS	GOALS
Friday			

	WORKOUT	MEALS	GOALS
Saturday			

	WORKOUT	MEALS	GOALS
Sunday			

Workout PLANNER

Week ______________________   *Month* ______________________

	WORKOUT	MEALS	GOALS
Monday			

	WORKOUT	MEALS	GOALS
Tuesday			

	WORKOUT	MEALS	GOALS
Wednesday			

	WORKOUT	MEALS	GOALS
Thursday			

	WORKOUT	MEALS	GOALS
Friday			

	WORKOUT	MEALS	GOALS
Saturday			

	WORKOUT	MEALS	GOALS
Sunday			

Workout PLANNER

Week ____________________   Month ____________________

	WORKOUT	MEALS	GOALS
Monday			

	WORKOUT	MEALS	GOALS
Tuesday			

	WORKOUT	MEALS	GOALS
Wednesday			

	WORKOUT	MEALS	GOALS
Thursday			

	WORKOUT	MEALS	GOALS
Friday			

	WORKOUT	MEALS	GOALS
Saturday			

	WORKOUT	MEALS	GOALS
Sunday			

Workout PLANNER

Week _______________________   Month _______________________

	WORKOUT	MEALS	GOALS
Monday			

	WORKOUT	MEALS	GOALS
Tuesday			

	WORKOUT	MEALS	GOALS
Wednesday			

	WORKOUT	MEALS	GOALS
Thursday			

	WORKOUT	MEALS	GOALS
Friday			

	WORKOUT	MEALS	GOALS
Saturday			

	WORKOUT	MEALS	GOALS
Sunday			

Workout PLANNER

Week ________________________ Month ________________________

	WORKOUT	MEALS	GOALS
Monday			

	WORKOUT	MEALS	GOALS
Tuesday			

	WORKOUT	MEALS	GOALS
Wednesday			

	WORKOUT	MEALS	GOALS
Thursday			

	WORKOUT	MEALS	GOALS
Friday			

	WORKOUT	MEALS	GOALS
Saturday			

	WORKOUT	MEALS	GOALS
Sunday			

Workout PLANNER

Week _______________________ *Month* _______________________

	WORKOUT	MEALS	GOALS
Monday			

	WORKOUT	MEALS	GOALS
Tuesday			

	WORKOUT	MEALS	GOALS
Wednesday			

	WORKOUT	MEALS	GOALS
Thursday			

	WORKOUT	MEALS	GOALS
Friday			

	WORKOUT	MEALS	GOALS
Saturday			

	WORKOUT	MEALS	GOALS
Sunday			

Workout PLANNER

Week ______________________   Month ______________________

	WORKOUT	MEALS	GOALS
Monday			

	WORKOUT	MEALS	GOALS
Tuesday			

	WORKOUT	MEALS	GOALS
Wednesday			

	WORKOUT	MEALS	GOALS
Thursday			

	WORKOUT	MEALS	GOALS
Friday			

	WORKOUT	MEALS	GOALS
Saturday			

	WORKOUT	MEALS	GOALS
Sunday			

Workout PLANNER

Week _______________________ *Month* _______________________

	WORKOUT	MEALS	GOALS
Monday			

	WORKOUT	MEALS	GOALS
Tuesday			

	WORKOUT	MEALS	GOALS
Wednesday			

	WORKOUT	MEALS	GOALS
Thursday			

	WORKOUT	MEALS	GOALS
Friday			

	WORKOUT	MEALS	GOALS
Saturday			

	WORKOUT	MEALS	GOALS
Sunday			

Workout PLANNER

Week _______________________   Month _______________________

	WORKOUT	MEALS	GOALS
Monday			

	WORKOUT	MEALS	GOALS
Tuesday			

	WORKOUT	MEALS	GOALS
Wednesday			

	WORKOUT	MEALS	GOALS
Thursday			

	WORKOUT	MEALS	GOALS
Friday			

	WORKOUT	MEALS	GOALS
Saturday			

	WORKOUT	MEALS	GOALS
Sunday			

Workout PLANNER

Week .... *Month* ....

	WORKOUT	MEALS	GOALS
Monday			

	WORKOUT	MEALS	GOALS
Tuesday			

	WORKOUT	MEALS	GOALS
Wednesday			

	WORKOUT	MEALS	GOALS
Thursday			

	WORKOUT	MEALS	GOALS
Friday			

	WORKOUT	MEALS	GOALS
Saturday			

	WORKOUT	MEALS	GOALS
Sunday			

Workout PLANNER

Week .... Month ....

	WORKOUT	MEALS	GOALS
Monday			

	WORKOUT	MEALS	GOALS
Tuesday			

	WORKOUT	MEALS	GOALS
Wednesday			

	WORKOUT	MEALS	GOALS
Thursday			

	WORKOUT	MEALS	GOALS
Friday			

	WORKOUT	MEALS	GOALS
Saturday			

	WORKOUT	MEALS	GOALS
Sunday			

Workout PLANNER

Week _______________   *Month* _______________

Monday	WORKOUT	MEALS	GOALS

Tuesday	WORKOUT	MEALS	GOALS

Wednesday	WORKOUT	MEALS	GOALS

Thursday	WORKOUT	MEALS	GOALS

Friday	WORKOUT	MEALS	GOALS

Saturday	WORKOUT	MEALS	GOALS

Sunday	WORKOUT	MEALS	GOALS

Workout PLANNER

Week .... Month ....

	WORKOUT	MEALS	GOALS
Monday			

	WORKOUT	MEALS	GOALS
Tuesday			

	WORKOUT	MEALS	GOALS
Wednesday			

	WORKOUT	MEALS	GOALS
Thursday			

	WORKOUT	MEALS	GOALS
Friday			

	WORKOUT	MEALS	GOALS
Saturday			

	WORKOUT	MEALS	GOALS
Sunday			

Workout PLANNER

Week _______________________   Month _______________________

Monday	WORKOUT	MEALS	GOALS

Tuesday	WORKOUT	MEALS	GOALS

Wednesday	WORKOUT	MEALS	GOALS

Thursday	WORKOUT	MEALS	GOALS

Friday	WORKOUT	MEALS	GOALS

Saturday	WORKOUT	MEALS	GOALS

Sunday	WORKOUT	MEALS	GOALS

HOW TO SCAN QR CODE

To scan a QR code, take the following general actions:

1. Open the Camera App: The majority of contemporary smartphones come with a built-in QR code scanning feature in their camera apps. Open the camera app on your smartphone.

2. Set the Camera Position: Slightly shake your phone and aim the camera toward the QR code you wish to scan. Verify that the well-lit QR code is inside the frame.

3. Scan the QR Code: The QR code ought to be instantly recognized by your smartphone's camera app. It could provide a link or a notification to access the content linked to the QR code.

4. Follow the Prompt: After the QR code is detected, adhere to any on-screen instructions. This could include clicking on a link to visit a website, downloading an application, or seeing particular content.

5. Access the Content : You ought to be able to view the content linked to the QR code after scanning it and following any instructions. This might be a website, an electronic voucher, contact details, or other kinds of information.

You might need to enable the QR code recognition option in your smartphone's settings or download a QR code scanning app from the app store if the camera app on your phone isn't picking up codes automatically. You should consult your device's user manual for more details since certain devices might have unique motions or instructions for reading QR codes.